The Distracted Centipede

...a Yoga experience

Mina Semyon

TRAFFORD

© Copyright 2004 Mina Semyon.
All rights reserved. No part of this publication may be reproduced, stored in a retrieval system, or transmitted, in any form or by any means, electronic, mechanical, photocopying, recording, or otherwise, without the written prior permission of the author.

Printed in Victoria, BC, Canada

Note for Librarians: a cataloguing record for this book that includes Dewey Decimal Classification and US Library of Congress numbers is available from the Library and Archives of Canada. The complete cataloguing record can be obtained from their online database at:
www.collectionscanada.ca/amicus/index-e.html
ISBN 1-4120-2926-0

TRAFFORD

This book was published *on-demand* in cooperation with Trafford Publishing. On-demand publishing is a unique process and service of making a book available for retail sale to the public taking advantage of on-demand manufacturing and Internet marketing. On-demand publishing includes promotions, retail sales, manufacturing, order fulfilment, accounting and collecting royalties on behalf of the author.

Offices in Canada, USA, UK, Ireland, and Spain
book sales for North America and international:
Trafford Publishing, 6E–2333 Government St.
Victoria, BC V8T 4P4 CANADA
phone 250 383 6864   toll-free 1 888 232 4444
fax 250 383 6804   email to orders@trafford.com
book sales in Europe:
Trafford Publishing (UK) Ltd., Enterprise House, Wistaston Road Business Centre
Crewe, Cheshire CW2 7RP UNITED KINGDOM
phone 01270 251 396   local rate 0845 230 9601
facsimile 01270 254 983   orders.uk@trafford.com
order online at:
www.trafford.com/robots/04-0754.html

10   9   8   7   6   5   4   3

Contents

Contents 3

Foreword 5

Acknowledgements 15

1. Distracted in a Ditch 21
2. What every centipede knows 32
3. A Yoga Story 39
4. Start by doing nothing 42
5. Don't hold your breath! 48
6. Pranayama: breathing exercises 55
7. More Yoga Stories 63
8. Yoga by e-mail: 70
9. All the things you can do lying on your back 73
10. Hips are for Swinging, Shoulders are for Shrugging 79
11. Yoga and Sex 90
12. Teaching and helping others 102
13. Still more Yoga stories 105
14. Life is not a technique or a series of crises 110
15. Awareness in everyday life 120

16.	Yoga and the Ageing Process	135
17.	...and still more Yoga Stories	141
18.	Take as long as it takes	148
19.	Letters from Students	152
20.	Gratitude to teachers past and present	158
21.	Take it with two pinches of salt	160
	Suggestions for further reading	163
	Resources	165

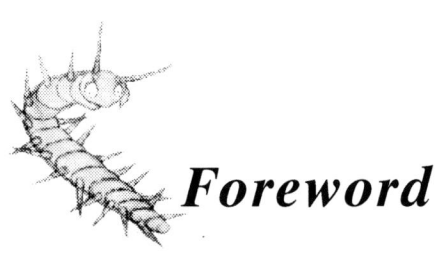
Foreword

by Dr Leon Redler, MD

*I*t gives me great pleasure to write a preface to this book. There are many books on Yoga available today which address our desire for health and fitness, lower stress levels, feeling well and looking good. This book delivers all that …and more. Moreover, it does so in a way that is fresh and timely, while faithful to the roots of ancient practice.

'The Distracted Centipede' is profoundly relevant to how we live our ordinary, everyday lives, and opens the possibility of transforming and uplifting the ordinary to the extraordinary without special techniques and without jumping on the bandwagon of yet another and latest healing fad, regimen or guru. There's an implicit assertion here, namely, that the ordinary is truly extraordinary and would be realised as such if only we, in the form of our habitual and distracted selves, could keep out of the way of that realisation. Mina shows a way to find all that is needed just where we are, acknowledging our relationship to the forces at play through and around us… and, in the course of that, being on course for relationships of greater ease, authenticity and responsibility with others.

It is a book that is meticulously honest, based on over thirty years of practice and teaching Yoga, but, at the same time on a life journey that has been no stranger to suffering and struggle. Mina starts each day, each lesson and each session of writing by trying to acknowledge where she is at, wherever that may be and whatever that may include of her thoughts, feelings and desires. And she invites, gently reminds and calls upon her students to do the same.

The points she makes are practical and down to earth as they are uplifting. She reminds us of basic issues that we need to 'take on board', such as:

(1) Acknowledge whatever is happening.
(2) Practise with an attitude of 'unknowing'.
(3) 'Let go' so as to open the way for wonder, discovering and fresh experiencing.
(4) Feel your contact with the ground and pull of gravity while ever releasing upward, skyward.
(5) Become aware and release anywhere in ones 'body-mind' where one is holding on or holding back, usually out of unrecognised and unacknowledged old and deep fear.
(6) Breathe mindfully and freely.

I first met Mina around 35 years ago. She had survived the hard and terrible conditions of the Second World War and of Russia under Stalin. By moving to South Africa and marrying Arthur Balaskas, she had found refuge and material comfort, but was still immersed in her own suffering, and, to a considerable extent, unavailable for others. She was, however, committed to find her way through and out of that prison and had a 'good nose' for those who embodied teachings that were relevant to her quest.

In London she was fortunate to meet Dr. R.D. Laing, perhaps the best known and controversial, psychiatrist–psychoanalyst–author of his day. She sought him as her guide.

In responding to her asking for his help and guidance, Ronnie Laing introduced her to Yoga and other eastern and western spiritual practices, consistent with his unwavering commitment to attending to body, mind and spirit, in the service of knowing oneself and radically alleviating suffering.

As I write these words, I am reminded of Mina telling me how, after she learned to stand on her head in the middle of the room, she'd find herself, while trying to keep her balance and, at the same time, silently reciting the Lord's Prayer, pondering the common ground between practising Yoga, being Jewish and the Christian prayer.

I saw Mina and her husband, some years later, on a BBC Television series on Yoga, 'Every Body Knows'. Mina was apparently able to practice and perform the most difficult yoga postures with ease. However, reflecting on that performance in later years, she told me how she realised her practice was 'still too superficial, too caught in appearances and not yet connecting with the source of physical, mental, emotional and spiritual well-being'.

What might that source be?

That question is worthwhile inquiring into and keeping in mind as one reads and practices in accord with the teachings of this book. It is through one's own inquiry and experience that deep and lasting benefit may be found.

Mina does not position herself as an expert, as 'the one who knows'. She values the position, or no-position, of 'unknowing', inspired by the 14th century (anonymously authored) text, "The Cloud of Unknowing," a text counselling loving God through a cloud of unknowing, and being open to the sanctity of the present moment. The yoga she teaches is not a mechanical practice or one meant to drive you to some imagined ideal of shape or fitness. In her yoga, as in any profound meditation, the musical metaphor of having the strings of your instrument not too loose and not too tight is an excellent one. Right effort is found by a relaxed mindfulness, honest acknowledgement of where one is and allowing the postures to unfold with the breath.

Mina gives high priority to our being mindful of our inspiration and expiration and to breathing freely. We can learn to allow and feel the breath of life move freely and deeply within us. We can let the in-breath come at the end of exhalation rather than grasping at it, allowing ourselves to be inspired and expired. In this way, we can be more in touch with birth and death in every moment.

On this way, we can become more aware of the wonder and impermanence of life and perhaps find the way to a breathing space that's light and free of fear and effort. In and on this way we can also let the other be the other, perhaps the best basis for love, friendship and the possibility of healing.

We are called to responsibility. And we can more responsibly respond to that call with a mindful and relaxed, and not 'uptight,' uprightness, one that nourishes humility, wonder, enjoyment, and the seeds of compassion rather than hatred and indifference.

What a difference such relaxed and responsible vigilance could make in our troubled world!

London 2004

Dr. Leon Redler is qualified in medicine, practices as a psychotherapist and is a member (and former Chair) of the Psychotherapy Training faculty of the Philadelphia Association, London. He is also co-director of The Mediation Partnership and of Just Listening and is qualified as a teacher of the Alexander Technique.

Andrew Feldmár, R. Psych., writes:

When Mina sent me the manuscript of her book 'The Distracted Centipede' I was reminded that I've known the authorless ditty, from which she borrowed, for many years, but until now I didn't realise its essential message:

> *The centipede was happy quite*
> *Until a toad in fun*
> *Said, 'Pray, which leg comes after which?'*
> *This raised her mind to such a pitch*
> *She lay distracted in a ditch*
> *Considering how to run.*

Every midwife, obstetrician, birth coach, all the experts who want to help women to give birth might do well to meditate upon these few lines of wise poetry. The martial arts, yoga, meditation, music, dance, and singing – all teach, transmit the same wisdom: GET OUT OF THE WAY!

Life knows how to bring new life into this world. Life knows how to protect itself. Life lives us. We are not surviving because of our cleverness and heroic efforts; we survive in spite of them. Faith is surrender to that which lives us.

Life knows how to walk the centipede; the self-conscious centipede doesn't.

Toad's question became a debilitating distraction.

Andrew Feldmár,
Vancouver 2004

Andrew Feldmár, R. Psych., is a psychologist practising psychotherapy in Vancouver, Canada, for the past 35 years now. He studied and worked with R. D. Laing from 1974 until Laing's death in 1989.
He writes and teaches internationally.

Igor Charkovsky - Water Birth pioneer in Russia writes about 'The Distracted Centipede'

Many books on Yoga are written in which the author hasn't always experienced the transformation this practice can bring in himself or herself. I am sorry to say that there are many books written by people who do not *feel* what they are writing.

I had the opportunity, the full value of which I didn't become aware of till later, of practising Yoga with Mina Semyon. During the lessons I realised that I hadn't known how to stand, or walk or sit down, or even lie down my whole life, because it turns out that all those activities are also an art. Suddenly I found out that I could move my body in ways I couldn't do 20 years ago - and I am already going into my sixth decade.

Because of the traumas left in me, for example, from sports injuries, the doctors said that my condition was very serious, predicting severe consequences. But after only three lessons, the pain in my hips and spine has disappeared. I even forgot about it, even though in the past I've tried to get rid of the pain by means of gymnastics, running etc.

Through practising with Mina I started to feel my energy gathering together.

The psychological problems, which made me feel pessimistic about certain projects, disappeared. What seemed impossible appeared possible after the Yoga lessons. My mind felt freer, lighter.

Many of the psychological problems that come from holding on to old family patterns - as they say - 'it runs in the family'; social patterns which seemed insurmountable and which I felt incapable of solving, seemed to drop away once I had come into a more harmonious state. I managed to come up with creative ideas for my own books. Many ideas, which had been dispersed, came together and became more convincing in my mind, after only a few lessons.

After a few hours of *pranayama* I started to see some events in my early childhood, which paralysed and slowed me down. After the Yoga I felt more empowered to deal with them. It brought my intellectual potential and clear vision to the forefront.

This allowed me to look from a high perspective at the things that a person who is at a lower level of energy finds impossible to deal with.

I had the opportunity to talk with some of Mina's other students and they told me that they were able to look differently at some of the psychological traumas they had experienced in childhood or even during the intra-uterine life.

The Yoga that Mina teaches allows one to return to the early stages of one's psychological and emotional development when different atmospheres, which became imprinted like ink into blotting paper, influenced one.

In my kind of work with newborn babies I can tell by the condition of the spine that at a certain stage of pregnancy the father fell in love with another woman. And that the baby seriously suffered from this situation, and felt divided because of the situation of conflict …and that experience got imprinted on the spine. Later, psychoanalysis confirms that this is what has happened. If all this gets worked through early in life, later the person will not have to go through all the love dramas.

When the body comes into order and harmony, the psychological life comes into harmony, and one begins to have clarity about and understanding of past suffering. The events that caused the trauma or phobia begin to be seen in a different light, and the person becomes healthy and robust, creativity awakens and is freed.

In Mina's book, *intuition* - developed over 30 years of working on herself to free herself from early traumas, thereby saving herself from patterns leading to depression and apathy, and moving to a higher level of creativity - is combined with *vision* gained as a result of the work on her body that helped to bring her psyche into an harmonious state. This is what she teaches to her students. Books can point the way, stimulate and inspire but only the individual can experience real understanding and deep feeling within.

This book is different from other books on the subject where Yoga postures are practised with a physical emphasis and without creating space for feeling the deep, subtle mechanisms that lie behind the postures and movements.

In Russia, where I work with pregnant women, I use *pranayama*, following and deepening the breath, which is a great method for bringing a woman's body into harmony with her baby inside her. As a result of Yoga and *pranayama* practice the problems of conflict get removed. In order to work in this way one needs subtle, deep intuitive vision of inner psychological mechanisms - something Mina Semyon possesses in abundance.

In Russia there are many old women seers, who can see the situations that caused difficulties such as stuttering, epilepsy, fears, bed-wetting and who, by praying, are able to remove such traumas. I had the opportunity to see this for myself. Such disturbances are connected with disturbances in meridians and different organs, and these old visionaries can heal such early traumas. But the work on one's body, clearing the meridians and bringing the interrelationship of all systems in the body into harmony through Yoga postures, is a way of healing yourself.

I know cases of healing, which were connected with hard work on one's body, which went on for a lifetime. In religious cultures there are fasts, prayer, systems of controlling the body and overcoming the animal levels and moving into high levels. So we need to work on the body to make it a temple for the soul and the spirit and not remain at the mercy of emotional structures lodged in it.

This work is very important for pregnant women to develop the capacity to communicate with the foetus and to understand the baby's emotional, psychological life. Such work would help people to reach deep realms of healing so as to heal the root of disturbances as early as in the womb.

This book will have a very important influence. I believe it would have great success in Russia and I would be glad to distribute it.

Igor Charkowsky

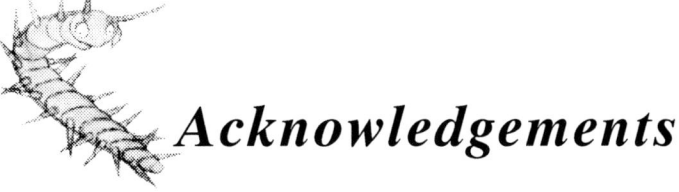
Acknowledgements

I would like to express my deepest gratitude to:

Ronnie Laing, my teacher and friend, who started me off on the voyage out of my wretched mind towards open heartedness and love.

Mary Ann Ephgrave, without whose patient and loving care, this book would not have seen the light of day.

Leon Redler for years and years of inspiring friendship through thick and thin, and for writing a heart-felt preface to my book.

Anthea Parashchak for her patience and wonderful talent in helping me to locate and start to bring out my real voice.

Hilmar Schonauer for helping me to get to know and trust myself.

Janet Balaskas for her warm friendship and encouragement over the years.

Dorothee Von Greiff for her loving friendship and support through all the vicissitudes of life.

Kevintao – for his music and Tango, from the stillness of Yoga into movement.

Dawn Mistress Tao for her computer magic.

Kate Levitt for her friendship and heartfelt accordion playing accompanying my Russian songs.

Jim Ephgrave for cooking the most delicious dinners and generally being a lovely presence while Mary Ann and I worked on the book.

Nick Hyams for his delightful drawing of The Distracted Centipede.

Hannah and Amy Redler for their love and friendship.

Edward Park for the photographs taken with such care and professionalism.

Sally Kohler for her boundless enthusiasm and generous support in sponsoring the publication of the book.

Andrew Feldmar for his wisdom, experience and many helpful suggestions.

Thanks to all my students for teaching me how to teach.

Thanks to the Friday group, which has met at my place for over ten years:

Paul McGuinnes, Kaoru, Nick Simons, Nick Hyams, Robbie Brook Howard, Alexis and Richard Pheiffer, for being a refuge, and oasis where one could 'just be' without any agendas, giving everyone a chance to heal and come closer to our authentic being.

And to all my friends, for their faith in me through all my struggles and doubts.

Thanks to all the publishers who refused my book proposals, as it helped to free my creative spirit from having to talk about how my book is different from other books on Yoga. There is a story about Beethoven, playing one of his sonatas to a small audience. When he had finished, someone asked, 'What is this sonata about?' In response Beethoven sat down and played it again. I feel this story will resonate in anyone involved in the creative process.

And as Alfred A. Tomatis said in his book, 'The Conscious Ear: My Life of Transformation Through Listening', 'There are no geniuses, some of us are just less damaged.'

This book is dedicated to my beautiful daughter and grandson, Kira and Alexi, with all my love.

'The centipede was happy quite
Until a toad in fun
Said, 'Pray, which leg comes after which?'
This raised her mind to such a pitch,
She lay distracted in a ditch,
Considering how to run.'

Anonymous

ONE

Distracted in a Ditch
How I came across Yoga

*We begin to glimpse the heart of the matter,
our childlike nature, kind, loving, and sensitive,
curious, trusting and playful.
We become true spiritual companions for each other.*

I was introduced to Yoga by R.D. Laing, the Scottish existentialist psychiatrist, poet, musician, and spiritual teacher while on holiday in Italy with our families in 1970. We stayed in a beautiful Palazzo by the sea with a private beach, ripe figs in the garden, a cook and a maid and I was feeling tired all the time.

I asked Ronnie, 'Why am I tired all the time?'

He replied, 'Have you heard of Yoga?'

I said, 'I heard about Yoga from a friend of Arthur's, (my husband at the time) who said that after practising Yoga for a year she started talking to trees and it made her grow taller.'

Ronnie suggested that we gather in the garden the following morning and he'd show us some Yoga postures. Early the next morning I went for a swim and a run on the beach to be in good shape for my first Yoga lesson. When I came back Ronnie was standing in the kitchen eating yesterday's ratatouille from the fridge and talking to Arthur about the Buddha's Four Noble Truths:

The truth of suffering
The origin of suffering: constant craving
The cessation of suffering: stopping the mind spinning
The path leading to the cessation of suffering: The Noble Eightfold Path

Ronnie spoke about the book by Nyanaponika Thera, '*The Heart of Buddhist Meditation*' and the four domains of mindfulness, which, he said, should be the foundation discipline for all therapists. The four domains are attentiveness to emotions, body posture, breathing and mental activities.

'The Buddha said, *To no other go for your light.* In other words', said Ronnie, 'get yourself together and be your own light. You can never realise this by thinking. It is in the region of unknowing …*agnosia*. Dionissius the Aeropogite said that *agnosia* is not ignorance, but rather the realisation that no finite knowledge can fully know the Infinite One. He is only truly approached by *agnosia* or that which is beyond and above knowledge.'

That day in the garden of the *Palazzo* is a very memorable day for me and one of the luckiest of my life. It was the first time I heard of the Buddha's teachings and yet Ronnie's words resonated with something deep within. I took to Yoga like a duck to water. I felt Yoga was going to save me in the nick of time. I found some postures easy and was inordinately proud of myself. Other postures I couldn't do and felt dejected. The only swinging I did in the 'swinging sixties' was from pride to dejection and back again. Like the guy on death row who was proud that his cell was bigger than the other guy's.

When Ronnie asked us to sit on the ground and take a deep breath I could only whimper with frustration. My chest was so tight I didn't know what a deep breath was. No wonder I was tired.

When we came back to London, sitting in a taxi at Heathrow I felt like Cinderella after the clock struck midnight, my ball gown turned into rags, the carriage into a pumpkin and the horses into mice. I felt that now I was going to lose being part of something meaningful, of real substance, that had come my way for the first time in my life that would take me beyond myself. Ronnie came up to the taxi and, as if reading my mind, asked, 'How would you like it if a group of us meets every morning to practice Yoga?' Would I?

We started meeting every morning at 7am and practising from BKS Iyengar's book *'Light on Yoga'*. We took turns being teacher by looking in the book and conferring whether the arm should be here or there, or the feet this or that angle.

Every week we took one new posture to learn. We discovered health shops, made our own yoghurt and had breakfast together after Yoga. What had started was a totally new experience of learning about ourselves and our relationship to each other, uncovering and releasing the childhood traumas and memories in the body, gradually getting glimpses of what lies beyond the conditioned mind.

Eventually we found a teacher and for two years had a two-hour lesson everyday. After the two years I felt I had shed the first layers of muscular armour.

My first "Aha" experience

Emotional pain was rising out of me like steam as a consequence of releasing my contracted body. I said to Ronnie: 'My life feels like a nightmare.'

He replied, 'It's easier to wake up from a nightmare than a pleasant dream.'

'Aha,' I thought, 'in this scheme of things I seem to have an advantage. If I'm in a nightmare, there is more incentive to wake up!'

I first read 'Yoga sutras' of Patanjali in 1970, and to this day still feel surprised and reassured that this ancient wisdom resonated in me before I even practised any Yoga or meditation.

I memorised the first nine sutras.

1. We now begin the exposition of Yoga
2. Yoga is controlling the activities of the mind

3. When mind is controlled self stays in his native condition
4. Otherwise he confirms to the nature of mind's activities
5. The activities are fivefold: some painful, others pleasurable
6. They are experience, perversion, delusion, sleep, recollection.
7. Control the activities by practice and detachment
8. Practice is effort towards concentration
9. Detachment is renunciation of all desire for objects seen or heard

When mind is controlled, self stays in his native condition.

I found it reassuring to discover that there is a *'native condition'* that doesn't depend on my social or cultural status and is beyond my conditioning. It seemed something could be done about all the disturbing emotions and thoughts that throw me off balance.

This *native condition* felt like a desirable place to get to know. How do we get there?

'Practice is effort towards concentration',

To this day, this is what I consider my own practice to be and this is what I am inspired to teach:
Effort towards concentration on
The breath,
Being present
Recognising how we disconnect
Letting go of thoughts or emotional reactions,
Connecting to gravity and letting the body release from the ground upwards.
Making a connection between feelings and the breath.

I got an email the other day with this amusing quote:

Practice makes perfect
Nobody is perfect
So why practise?

True? As my mother used to say 'Every joke has a grain of truth in it.' But then an interview with the Great Russian pianist Vladimir Horowitz comes to mind. When asked how much he practised he replied, 'I never practise, I play at home and when the time comes I get transported to the concert hall and continue playing.'

This is how I understood this sutra;

'Practice is effort towards concentration' …it is mindfulness of every moment of everyday life. Practise and playing are not separate.

'Detachment is renunciation of all desire for objects seen or heard',

Now this one I had a real problem with. I couldn't even begin to allow a little chink of light between my attachments and letting go of them. I didn't even know that such a thing existed. 30 odd years later what do I understand by *'letting go of desire for objects seen or heard?'* How do you renounce all desire?

Well, sometimes I detect a nagging sensation inside that is making me feel uneasy, edgy. If I stop, slow down, become quiet, take a breath, I am able to identify what is behind this vague unease. It is craving, *wanting*. My whole being is reaching out for something from someone who is not here. Maybe it is the child's desire for comfort and safety that went unfulfilled.

Having recognised what it is, I make a feeling contact with the craving and feel my breath releasing. I say to myself, 'Relax, you will survive without this response you crave so much, the craving has become a habit and you have locked the habit and lost the key. The *key* is your awareness, this capacity to turn within and shine some light on it.'

Identifying the energy of craving helps to connect up with the core of your being, the greatest security and nourishment there is. Suddenly you feel there is nothing missing, wholeness is within you. Learning to take care of this needy, craving inner child will help you develop compassion and the capacity to take care of others.

Letting go is loosening the grip and allowing the breath to flow freely and rhythmically. Letting go is a profound position of trust in life, becoming an active agent rather than a passive victim. Loving, rather than wanting to be loved.

To accept is to go with what's happening at this moment and respond spontaneously. To resist means to cut off and react to the present situation with familiar, conditioned, 'safe' responses. Letting go improves your health. When the fruit is ripe the tree surrenders it. When our mental and physical habits have become redundant we can consciously surrender them like ripe fruit.

All I know is that those moments when I manage to let go of the tyranny of constant craving are the most profound moments of peace I know. It feels like releasing a muscle and all the strain of 'having to keep it all together' disappears. Why can't I be in that place always? It seems I have to keep on going through whatever obscures this place again and again and keep touching it afresh. We talk about high consciousness, but by doing inner work first of all we become conscious of how things *are*, which may not always be to our taste.

First we have to be able to detect the presence of constant craving inside, wanting what you don't have, not wanting what you have. If you really allow yourself to feel it, it feels like hell, there is nowhere to hide from it. You can try to distract yourself, watch a movie, go out for a meal, go shopping, but the *craving* will return. Nothing satisfies this monster.

It is the nature of desire; it doesn't matter what and how much you have, you can still want more. I once knew a man who said he envied me my capacity to want because he never got a chance to want anything. Every time a new toy appeared at the famous New York 5th Avenue toyshop, his father had it delivered to his already toy-filled room. I never had any toys, yet the story is the same.

So what is the answer? To call it's bluff, to recognise the craving for what it is, to cultivate the skilful means of letting it go. It takes time and practice. There is a Russian saying, *It takes a lot of milk to make a little cream.* I used to fear that by letting go of craving I'd turn into a dried out, indifferent and undesirable prune. But gradually I realised that the state of mind of craving stands in the way of being fully alive.

When I first read

the activities of the mind are five-fold, some painful, others pleasurable

I thought, 'So it means that whether we are in pain or pleasure there is a need to control the activities of the mind.'

Somehow it felt like a great leveller. There was a place to be that wasn't dependent on passing experiences whether pleasant or unpleasant. I notice that sometimes I sit and observe my breath and feel emotional or physical pain, other times I sit and observe my breath and experience pleasure, but the centre remains the same. You can be beside yourself with pain or with pleasure.

What a relief! No need to be at the mercy of moods. No matter what the circumstances there is a choice as to how you respond. Not easy, but possible. That's all I know for now and for that I am grateful, when I remember to remember to be grateful. As William Blake said, '*Gratitude itself is Heaven*'.

Practise of Yoga positions, or *asanas*, with mindfulness of breathing, gradually enables us to become conscious of the tensions in our body and of our habitual ways of holding the body, and teaches a discipline of becoming aware of how the body functions in relationship to gravity. It also makes us more aware of how the condition of the body relates to our mental and emotional habits. The practice helps to develop skills to deal with the emotional patterns that get revealed as the result of letting go. We can't let go of that of which we are not aware.

The spirit in which we inhabit our body is expressed in our body language. 'Uptight' literally means being tight in the upper regions of the body. If you are pulled up into your shoulders and neck you are weak in your centre of gravity. Painful experiences can create defensive tensions that prevent us from being in touch with who we really are.

We say, 'It runs in the family!' But it only runs in the family because we don't question it. We need to get the grannies out of our groins, the centuries of inhibition and prohibition that sit there, stopping us from inhabiting our bodies with ease. The ultimate trust is to let go, stop controlling the body and allow for the experience of wholeness to awaken.

When we establish a relationship with the body's innate wisdom, trust awakens in the body's self-healing capacity. Often conventional medicine ignores the body's natural capacity for healing, striving to get rid of symptoms before reading their meaning.

Hatha Yoga, the physical-mental aspect of yoga, is a preparation for Yoga becoming a way of life - physically, mentally, ethically and spiritually. I feel that in order to get to our common ground as fellow human beings we have to get in touch with, acknowledge, accept and let go of, our particular, individual ways of holding on to our defences. By starting to melt these structures we begin to glimpse the heart of the matter, our childlike nature, kind, loving, sensitive, curious, trusting and playful. We become true spiritual companions for each other.

Yoga helped me to survive Stalin and a Jewish mother.

I was born on the border of Russia and Poland before the Second World War. The border was in a constant state of change. A story went around about this guy whose house was right on the border. When the Russian authorities came to change it they asked the guy, 'Where do you want to be – in Russia or in Poland?' The guy screwed his eyes up to the sky and said 'Oh, in Poland – I couldn't take another Russian winter!' For telling a story like that one could end up in a Siberian hard labour camp during the Stalinist purges, labelled an anti-Soviet agitator.

When, years later, my mother and I left Russia and ended up in Cape Town, South Africa, at the height of the apartheid era, from the frying pan into the fire, I was in a lot of emotional pain, resulting, amongst other things, in crying every day. In those days

I thought that crying everyday was a normal thing everyone did like brushing teeth and having breakfast.
My mother asked, 'Why are you crying?'
'I am worried.'
'Here, have a *Librium.*'
'I don't want tranquillisers – I want to live.'
'Akh – don't be a silly girl, there is plenty of time for that. In the mean time take a Librium. I take one a day and' – pointing to the table, 'is this table worried? That's how much I am worried!'

Well, I didn't want to be like that table. I didn't want to be dulled by tranquillisers. I wanted to feel fully alive by getting through the pain, although I didn't yet know how. So when Ronnie Laing introduced me to yoga and mindfulness I felt hopeful that there was a way of touching and releasing the traumas lodged in my mind and body.

Through the practice of yoga and mindfulness I gained a sense of what is truly essential. Thankfully I never had an inclination to speculate on whether I was born before and whether I will be born again or whether or not there is such a thing as reincarnation. All I notice is that how I think, speak and behave affects my life here and now and how I 'incarnate' into the next moment. And there *is* something I can do about it. I became less concerned about what other people think of me, they'll think of something else in a minute. Being *authentic* became more important than being *good.*

> *Authentic – an emotionally appropriate, significant, purposive, and responsible mode of human life: New Oxford Dictionary.*

I feel that being *authentic* has to be good for our individual and collective well being. I somehow don't think that in primitive tribes teenagers need to rebel, because what they learn from adults is sensible training for living life. What our teenagers see is often so twisted and disconnected that when they start thinking for themselves they want to get away from it as far as possible. I once saw a picture of a girl with rings pierced through her lips, tongue and nostrils, razor blades in her ears, hair orange, pink and green and the caption said, 'I survived a Jewish mother!'

I felt suffocated by my mother's beliefs and the conditioning that she tried to impose on me out of her fear and ignorance. But at the same time I clung to her because I was brainwashed to believe that I couldn't survive without her. It took 30 odd years of Yoga, therapy, fasts and brown rice diets to change the chemistry of this attachment.

But the most fundamental change is connecting to my innermost being that is beyond differences, my own connection to the life source without intermediaries.

Asanas

The fact that I first heard about Yoga from Ronnie Laing in the context of my wishing to be released from the grip of my past had a profound effect on my subsequent approach to practise and teaching. It became apparent to me that psychotherapy and being listened to and acknowledged, however deeply and meaningfully, were not enough to change deeply ingrained habits of mind and body and to heal the wounds. I also needed a discipline to help me get in touch with all the old restrictive patterns in my mind and body and gradually learn to live without them. Practise of Yoga and mindfulness became this discipline.

I've already mentioned that a group of us started practising from *'Light on Yoga'* by B.K.S.Iyenger, taking turns reading out the instructions of a posture and conferring as to whether arms should be at this or that angle. For six months we did this without a teacher. It did us no harm although having said that, there was a queue of us at the osteopath's every Monday morning!

My personal feeling is that you can't really learn asanas from a book without a teacher's individual instruction. I would, however, like to express what are to me the basic principles that need to be applied to practising asanas, whether the postures are sitting, standing, lying down or inverted. These principles, the 'royal jelly' of the practice, are not limited to 'yoga' but need to be applied in daily life as well.

1. The body doesn't need our interference. It needs our presence. Presence makes sure that you allow your breath to flow; that you feel contact with the ground; that you imagine space inside your body. Presence notices if the mind wanders off. It's not 'flowery talk', if you use your imagination you can experience the body unfolding like a flower. Every posture is a prayer.

2. Continuous mindfulness of our relationship to gravity.

3. Realising that the greatest antidote to stress is awareness of the spine elongating in two directions: down to the ground and releasing upwards toward the sky.

4. Allowing the left and right sides to communicate.

5. Awareness of how our thoughts and emotions effect our breathing and learning to release and calm the breath through all the disturbances that arise.

6. Realizing the need to release the neck and allow the head to find its balance on top of the broad base of the atlas.

7. Not to hold your breath for anything or anybody.

8. To 'remember to remember' to apply all these principles in daily life.

When we surrender all the tensions and grasping and connect to the vital energy we are in a state of prayer.

TWO

What every centipede knows

The body doesn't need our interference;
it is a unified system to which we can safely surrender
if we let go of holding on for dear life.

*T*he centipede is 'programmed' to be a centipede; it simply can't deviate or go astray. It doesn't need workshops on how to deal with the complexity of all its legs, provided that it doesn't get distracted 'by a toad'. Human beings do get distracted therefore more can go wrong with the human being than the centipede. By becoming distracted we become fragmented and lose the sense of our unified being.

To live in that place of deep connectedness requires being present and aware at every moment. Of all living creatures only human beings resist and deny the need for being present and aware.

Distracted by what?

>Fear
>Anger
>Greed
>Craving
>Envy
>Jealousy
>Arrogance
>Pride

> Praise
> Blame
> What other people think of you
> You name it

Disconnected from what?

> From being whole, being present and aware.
> From love in our hearts.

Aware of what?

> Of the breath as it comes and goes
> Contact with the ground as you sit, stand, walk or lie down
> Aware of the body grounded and infinitely releasing upwards
> Aware of thoughts and the way they create emotional weather
> Of likes and dislikes, dissatisfaction or satisfaction
> Wishing to possess, to hold on.

Often what we call 'health' is really just a habit we got used to!

Slow down, become still, and listen within. How do you feel?

I ask a student, 'How are you?' 'Fine,' she says, with a bright smile on her face. We do some breathing and relaxing. After a while she says, 'I didn't realise how heavy my head feels and I have pain in my shoulders.'

'How are you really?' I ask.

'Oh, I have a new job. I need an office and they say there isn't a spare room available and it's all just too much. That's why I'm feeling like this – I'm just stressed out.'

'It seems to me that these days 'stressed out' has become a way of evading how we really feel. 'Stressed' is a symptom of emotional illiteracy. But the body doesn't lie. Suppressed emotions and thoughts are expressed in the body in all sorts of ways. If we start paying attention and learn to connect with our thoughts and feelings in an 'embodied' way we'll start taking responsibility for them and at least take a pause before blaming them on the circumstances or other people. Feelings that aren't connected to the breath become concretised and dumped into the body. Much of our illness is really blockage of energy. True health lies in being able to be in touch with our feelings by staying connected to the breath and letting go of unnecessary tensions.

She became quiet. 'How do I feel? That's a very good question.'

What does it mean – to relax; to be 'relaxed'?

> ***relaxed:*** free from tension and anxiety; at ease. (*New Oxford Dictionary*)
> ***ease:*** in Latin, means ***elbows akimbo***, having elbowroom.

Oh, to be at ease!

To relax consciously we need first to become aware of and acknowledge that we are not relaxed. Ease comes from being grounded, with the mind, body and breath balanced and in tune. Anxiety is the result of cutting off feelings in the present moment. Suppressed feelings and emotions create tension that can lead to mental imbalance and physical dis-ease. Most of the time we don't realise that we are suppressing our feelings. But if we get into the habit of paying attention to them, acknowledging and releasing them, and at the same time connecting to our breathing, we could heal ourselves *before* a physical or emotional crisis develops. For me the only time I can say I am truly relaxed and not a danger to myself or others is when I am in a state of acceptance, even acceptance of my non acceptance.

If you become aware of your breathing right now you'll probably realise that you are holding your breath!

Become quiet and tune into your breath. Slow down. Drop your shoulders. Let your energy flow. Imagine the rhythm of a growing plant. It will allow your bodily functions to flow more freely. When mind, body, breath and heart come into union we start to feel whole.

Become aware of how you waste energy by blocking the breath. This is what affects the healthy functioning of the organs of the body. Organs would interact harmoniously, like instruments in an orchestra, if the body were free of unnecessary tensions.

The more aware we are of our inner body, the deeper our relaxation will be on a visceral level. The more we are truly present in our body and aware of how thoughts, feelings and outside conditions affect it, the more we are able to let go of unnecessary tensions. If we are tired we can get behind our tiredness to the source of energy that is behind tiredness. We might still be tired, but relaxed with it.

The moment we let go, energy begins to flow and we find ourselves present in the *'now'*. We let life in. We arrive at this *'now-ness'* by gentle attentiveness to the details of our ordinary activities. We can invoke magic in our bodies through this awareness. No matter what our age or physical defects we can still experience unity in our bodies and communication between our head, neck, shoulders, arms, legs, feet, hips, genitals.

When we feel connected our bodies express friendliness towards our environment and ourselves. There is a harmony in the way we sit, stand, walk, lie down and speak that affects our health, physical as well as emotional, and the way we affect others. By gradually letting go of our habitual ways of holding on we begin to realise that joy doesn't depend on the circumstances of our lives, it rises out of an open heart. And sometimes it has to reach crisis point before we start paying attention. But no experience, if we learn from it, is a waste of time; it takes as long as it takes to wake up.

Yoga is not about *getting there;* it's about *being here.*

I remember how once, when I experienced a moment of what felt like 'presence', I wanted to hold on to it and be in the same state of mind later on, when I met up with a friend. Then I had another insight; *'You don't need to hold on; if you can be here now, you'll be able to be there then.'* For one moment I saw clearly that the place from which I experience presence is always here, it is a matter of connecting up to it, 'it' is the 'source', like the electricity current. The following story illustrates it beautifully.

An avid student of Buddhism would often discuss the teachings with a Master who lived across the river. One day the student felt inspired and wrote the following poem:

> I bow my head to the heaven within heaven
> Hairline rays illuminating the universe
> The eight winds cannot move me
> Sitting still upon the purple golden lotus.

Impressed by himself, the student dispatched somebody to deliver this poem to the Master. He felt certain that the Master would be just as impressed, maybe even recognise his enlightenment.

The "eight winds" in the poem referred to praise, ridicule, honour, disgrace, gain, loss, pleasure and misery - interpersonal forces of the material world that drive and influence the hearts of men. The student was saying that he had attained a higher level of spirituality, where these forces no longer affected him.

Smiling, the Master wrote, "FART" on the manuscript and had it returned to the student across the river.

Expecting compliments and a seal of approval, the student was shocked when he saw what the Master had written.

He hit the roof, "How dare he insult me like this? Why that lousy old Master! He's got a lot of explaining to do!"

Full of indignation, the student got into a boat and ferried himself to the other shore as quickly as possible. Once there, he jumped off and charged into the hut where the Master lived. He wanted to find the Master and demand an apology.

He found the Master's door closed. On the door was a piece of paper, with the following two lines:

> 'The eight winds cannot move me,
> One fart blows me across the river'.

Penetrate to the present moment.

If you live in the past, the best part of you is underground, like a root vegetable!

In order to live in the present we have to understand, accept and let go of the pain connected with the past. This is not a matter of obsessively digging into the past. Just by paying attention to the present we can become aware of how the past still lives on in the memory of our muscles, nerves and cells, coursing through the blood, preventing us from living life to our full potential now.

In the practice of Yoga we always have to start from the beginning. Whether we've been practising for a long time or have only just started, it is always a matter of connecting to where we are at this present moment mentally, emotionally, and physically and starting from there.

The practice of Yoga is an open invitation to the present moment. The present moment is always here to return to, however far we've wandered off. It is closer to us than our breath. Like the sun penetrating through the clouds, so we too can penetrate through all the noise and restlessness in the mind-body to stillness.

> *'Nothing in all creation is so like God as Stillness'*
> *Meister Eckhart*

The body doesn't need our interference; it is a unified system to which we can surrender if we let go of holding on for dear life. The spine will release upwards if we let it because that is how it is meant to be ...upright, not uptight, grounded in the base and releasing upwards.

But if we are not in touch with this two-way movement then it's an effort to have to keep the body up, because it's in conflict, fighting against the natural forces. To be in touch with the Divine is also about being in touch with the Divine in our bodies. What does it mean? It means to be in touch with the forces that govern the body. Every tree, every animal *knows* it. Only human beings are capable of perverting it, imposing a false balance, a twisted security. So we need to return, to get in touch with our innate balance again and again, not as an idea but as real life experience in the body. This is what I feel passionate about and is my book's special message.

Yoga practised with mindfulness of breathing can help us become aware of and look deeper into how we get distracted. It can help us to keep on returning to awareness and presence.

This book is about how I got to 'here' from 'there'. 'Here' is where I got smart — figured out that the present moment is where guilt and blame, pride and shame, fear and hate have no breeding ground – the only place where the buggers can't get you! 'There' is where I lay, *Distracted in a ditch, considering how to live'*, in the grip of early painful memories – from which there seemed to be no escape. The best definition of meditation I've come across is:

'Meditation means to live without being distracted.'

THREE

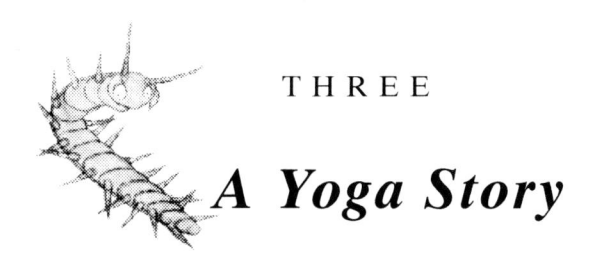

A Yoga Story

'I can't sleep, can't relax.'

A very endearing, tall and bulky orthodox Jewish man comes for a Yoga lesson. He tells me that he has six children, all boys, and another on the way. Oy vey!

He says he can't relax, can't sleep, and doesn't understand why.

I ask him to lie down on the floor with knees bent, feet in line with his hips, heels a little wider than his toes, in order to broaden and relax the lower back.

'It's not easy,' he says.

I say, 'Don't worry, it's safe, you can't fall off the floor.'

He laughs, and can't stop laughing, his feet like jumping beans.

Eventually he settles down, he is lying relatively still. I hold his feet down for a while to show him what it feels like to have his feet in line and grounded. Before I can say another word, I hear he's fallen fast asleep. I let him sleep. I sit and observe my breath.

After a while I say, 'Now gently open your eyes.' He opens his eyes.

His face lights up in an amazed grin, 'I fell asleep!'

'Yes, you did. Now, roll over to one side, stand up and let's have a look at your standing posture.'

He stands up, his feet wide apart, heels in, toes out, pelvis pushed forward, chin sticking out, the spinal curves in disarray.

I say, 'Let's start from your feet. Have a good look at your feet.'

'Look at my feet? What's so interesting about my feet?' says his disarming smile.

'The feet need to be *grounded* for the spine to feel supported free and released.

Imagine your feet are like the roots of a tree going deep down into the earth and the top of the tree is free, infinitely growing upwards. Imagine your upper body supported from the base becoming infinitely open to the sky. Close your eyes, relax your breath and become aware of your feet touching the ground.'

I see his feet jumping outwards.

I say, 'Let your feet become quiet. Do nothing, just feel the contact your feet are making with the ground.'

His grin gets even broader, 'How do I feel the feet in contact with the ground?'

'How do you feel when someone touches you?'

'Ah!'

He closes his eyes, and concentrates with all his might. His feet stay straight but now his eyes are all tight.

I say, 'Relax your eyes.' He laughs. His eyes relax but his feet shoot outwards again.

We keep quiet for a while,

'Now put your feet parallel, in line with your hips, your heels a little wider than your toes.'

He looks bemused. I help him to put his feet straight. He looks with wonder at his feet as if they performed a miracle. A second later they jump again to their habitual position.

I say, 'Look again; this position of the feet does not give any support to your spine. Just take notice of it and put your feet back into the parallel position. Does it feel different?'

He does so, stays for a moment and his feet shoot back yet again into the habitual position. I start laughing, he joins in, and we laugh and laugh.

I say, 'This is a good demonstration of the power of habit.'

He laughs, 'Sure is.'

FOUR

Start by doing nothing

*The entry into your being is through
what is happening at this moment.*

Stop and become quiet. Listen. Most of us have a lot of noise going on in our heads, which we wish we could stop. 'Why did I say that? I wish I hadn't. Why didn't she call me? She never calls me; I always call her. The world is a mess, so what's the point? Life is unfair. I wish I could live by the sea...' and before you know it you're in a spin.

Your muscles respond to all your thoughts and emotions if you are not conscious of the process. Your shoulders go up to your ears, your chest becomes tight, you clench your jaw, your neck becomes rigid and pretty soon you're exhausted and don't know why. All that wasted energy!

I once spent a whole year being jealous of a non-existent female harp-player!

My partner, a musician and composer, told me in a moment of inspiration, that he had decided to put a harp into his composition. Instantly, like lightening, I was inflamed by jealousy. I saw this harp player, a beautiful young woman, her exquisite fingers plucking the strings. I'd wake up at night racking my brain whether I'd ever seen a male harp player. No! They are normally women! In the end he decided to take the harp out...

Sometimes the noise in the head reaches unbearable proportions. You can't stop it by using willpower. I find this mindfulness exercise helpful:

Aware of the activities in my mind I breathe in.
Aware of the activities in my mind I breathe out.

By acknowledging the activities they begin to calm down and you become aware that there *is* stillness at the centre of the storm.

How I spent the night with jealousy.

H. didn't ring and didn't come that evening. I couldn't make contact with him either. He had spent every night with me for a year or so. My mind was in a spin; 'He is with another woman.'

I was supposed to be giving a workshop on Yoga and Mindfulness the following morning with L. In the grip of jealousy I felt what a fraud I was going to feel the next day, talking about mindfulness and observing our thoughts and emotions, letting them go and bringing attention to our breathing. And besides I'd be tired as I was unable to sleep. I told myself that the workshop would be a failure. I tossed and turned and made cups of tea waiting for the phone to ring. I tried to practice mindfulness; 'Ok, acknowledge your thoughts, *he is with another woman*, and breeeeeathe in, *he is with another woman* and breeeeeathe out,' but the grip of jealousy in my solar plexus wouldn't go away. I prayed, 'Please don't let me be a fraud.'

Then I thought, 'OK, I want to be with him but my companion for the night is jealousy. Hello jealousy, we are going to spend the night together. I feel jealous and I breathe in, I feel jealous and I breathe out.' I surrendered to jealousy and finally fell asleep. In the morning I woke up still feeling jealous but I didn't feel a fraud. I thought, 'I'm not claiming perfection, I'm practising mindfulness to the degree of which I am capable at this moment. I feel jealousy but I am not beside myself with jealousy.' Intimacy with jealousy helped me to maintain presence.

Slow is not lethargic

In the film *'Zorba the Greek'* the English writer tells Zorba how he watched a butterfly emerging from a cocoon. Wanting to hurry up the process, he held the fragile creature in his hands and started blowing on it. The butterfly came out all crumpled up and soon died. Heartbroken, he resolved never to interfere again in the natural process of unfolding.

The most fundamental trust, I think, is in letting go of feeling that we have to control our bodies. If we are in touch with our natural centre of gravity we realise that there is nothing to hold on to and no need to hold on. Easier said than done. I experience the letting go in moments, yet the fear to totally let go keeps returning. Have you heard the one about the guy who fell off a cliff and just managed to hold on to a branch? So there he is, hanging onto the branch. Below is an abyss and above, the rock he can't get back onto.

So he prays, 'Is there anyone up there? Please help me.'

A voice replies, 'Yes, I am here, just let go and my arms will be there to catch you.'

The guy thinks for a moment and then says, 'Is there anybody else up there?'

In the body it is unarguable that making contact and establishing a steady connectedness to the ground connects you with freedom and stability. Continuous practice and experience of this connectedness awakens the confidence to keep letting go of holding on to the old tensions and stresses.

Scientists say that *excessive motor-activity of the body is responsible for the neurological diseases of our age.* Our own experience tells us that slowing down and feeling the flow of life in our body naturally slows down wear and tear and allows the body to heal itself. Slow does not mean passive or lethargic. The unfolding of a flower is slow and full of vitality and direction.

Connect to your own rhythm
Whatever you are doing - do less, strain less.

To claim the right to be genuinely at ease, in touch with the still centre within, is not as simple as it sounds. Our social conditioning is based on having to be 'stressed out'. If you are listening to someone who is distressed and stay calm yourself it may appear to them that you don't care. In order to show how much we care we seem to think that we have to demonstrate that we are listening intently by looking intense and not allowing ourselves to relax. A bit like passing a driving test when the important thing seems to be that we make sure the examiner sees us looking in the rear view mirror a lot, rather than how safe and relaxed our driving is.

You can be relaxed *and* responsive and caring at the same time. You don't need to get a stiff neck to show how much you care. In fact the more relaxed you are inside, the less you are 'doing', the more you are able to be truly present, to listen and to hear.

I once asked Ronnie Laing, 'How come you sometimes don't answer when I ask you a question?'

He replied, 'I don't like to interrupt myself.'

The body is potentially like a well conducted orchestra, with all the organs functioning in connection with each other, in perfect harmony and rhythm. The less we are 'doing' and interfering, the more in touch we become with our inner rhythm, our own experience of the pulse of life.

When we are out of touch with the pulse of life, we feel discontented, restless and anxious. We might try too hard to please other people, frightened of being rejected if we don't play their song and dance.

There is exquisite pleasure in the luxury of feeling free to follow your own rhythm, reclaiming it from the cacophony of the conditioned emotional noise. To be in tune with your *biorhythm* is the greatest gift.

'Yoga is too slow for me'

At Hampstead Heath Ladies' pond I overheard two women talking:

'Oh, you look so beautiful, I didn't think it was you!'

'Yes, I've just been on holiday. How are you?'

'Oh, stressed out'

'Maybe you should try Yoga'.

'I do Pilates, I hate Yoga, it's too slow, too stationary, I hate all the talk about going inside, going within.'

Yes, there is a common misconception that slowing down, going within, means becoming obsessively introspective.

Could it be fear of finding out what lies beneath the 'stressed out' state, opening Pandora's box? But there is no truly effective way of becoming free of stress except by going right into and through what lies behind it. And there isn't a once and for all clean up, it's an on-going process of being aware and present.

So you can go as fast or as slow as you want as long as you are in rhythm with your organism. But in order to get in touch with that rhythm we do need to slow down

'Life is so short we must move very slowly.'
A Thai saying

'Right effort'

'Right effort' is one of the fruits of continuous practice of Yoga. It is a way of practising Yoga postures without straining. In right effort there is no stress. Becoming aware of the two-way movement of the spine and keeping this awareness in every position is the best antidote to stress I know of. It means letting go of everything that blocks the grounding and lengthening of the spine and the flow of the breath.

Of course, we can't even begin without some effort, but we gradually learn from experience what is wrong effort and how it stands in the way of unfolding. *'Wrong effort'* is straining, trying too hard, disconnecting from breathing, using will power to 'achieve' a posture, wanting to be 'good' at Yoga.

> Lie on your back with your feet on the floor, knees bent, feet in line with your hips, heels a little wider than the toes.
> Give yourself a big hug, do a little wriggle and open the space between the shoulder blades.
> Let go of your wrists and let your hands hang loose.
> Do nothing.
> When we say 'do nothing' we become aware of how much we are doing! It can be quite amusing to imagine a camera that can see inside your mind and all the turmoil going on in there while you are lying on the floor

seemingly peaceful. Acknowledge what is happening in your mind. Give yourself a lot of space with all your feelings and thoughts and current inner weather. Accept everything as it is, just for now. Notice how after a while your breathing begins to relax and expand all by itself. Now you might be able to distinguish your thoughts, which were a general anxious blur before. You might feel a momentary release of the strain of having to keep it all together.

Connect to your breathing as it is, do nothing, let the breath do what it wants to do.

Observe the sensations accompanying your breathing, either in the lower abdomen or in the nostrils as the air enters and leaves. Notice thoughts as they arise, observe them, don't follow them; bring your awareness back to watching the breath.

Notice how after a while, by slowing down and making deeper contact with your inner rhythm, you experience the stillness within. Become aware of how easily the mind can get stirred up by thoughts and how the practice of slowing down and becoming mindful of the breath can bring it back to the stillness. If you can bear to stay with your disturbances you'll learn how to quieten your random thoughts with rhythmical breathing. And so we gradually become more and more familiar with that place of being present honouring the moment and being open to what it has to offer.

'At the still point,
there is the dance'
T.S.Elliot

FIVE

Don't hold your breath!

> *Inspire* – *breath, courage, vigour, the soul, life, to breathe, to infuse life into breathing, to have an animating effect upon, to cause, guide, communicate, or motivate as by divine or supernatural influence.*
> Webster's New World Dictionary

Holding the breath is a short-term strategy for not feeling.

Why is it that we have a problem about being sensible when it comes to nourishing ourselves? Why wouldn't we want to take care of ourselves and stop being self-destructive? Maybe it's because we are still stuck in the infantile stage of wanting care because we never got it in the first place. If you never got enough of the right quality of caring you could be stuck in an unconscious attitude of 'why should I care if they didn't?', cutting off your nose to spite our face and not being aware of it. Unless we can get in touch with our feelings and allow ourselves to fully grieve for the love that wasn't there our resentment cannot transform into forgiveness. Then we continue being emotional cripples, longing to be loved and being unable to love.

'How can I change this pattern?'

By practising being mindful of thoughts and emotional structures, being honest that some of those patterns are like a stuck record playing the same old tune over and over again.

Meditate on the difference between feelings and emotional reactions. Feelings are not the same as emotional reactions. You can feel whatever it is that you are feeling and stay connected to yourself and your dignity. If you are unable, at the moment, to express your feelings to others, you can start by expressing them to yourself. You can listen to yourself the way you'd like to be listened to. A 'feeling' is a 'response'; an 'emotion' is a 'reaction'. Staying with your feelings and not losing your connection is what is called ***presence***. If you get caught up in an emotional reaction you lose your presence.

Stay with your breath. Observe your thoughts and feelings, acknowledge them, let them be and return to the breath. If you are feeling bored observe the boredom, let it be and return to the breath.

No matter how much stretching we do, or how many massages we get and how wonderful we feel at the time, it doesn't last. What is lasting and always available is being mindful at every moment, mindful of your body, thoughts, speech and breath and connecting to the love in your heart.

Sit comfortably on a cushion. Let your sacrum release to the ground. Let your shoulder blades be free like wings. Enjoy the sensation of breathing and of life breathing you. Being present and aware can become our constant companion no matter where we are and what we are doing.

Breathing in and breathing out can be akin to receiving and giving. To let this process become more harmonious can be a lifetime's task, but since it is the most important component of physical and mental health, what better way to occupy our time? Imagine the flow of your breath expanding your energy and opening the pathways to joy.

If you observe a little baby breathing it becomes very clear that the baby is *being breathed*; one can see the diaphragm working. Imagine being free, your breathing happening all by itself without interference.

Begin by paying attention to your next few breaths. It is possible to do whatever you are doing and notice your breath at the same time. Feel the quality of each inhalation, feel the parts of your body that move or don't move with each in and out breathe.

As you read this page, notice the wave of your breathing, your unique rhythm, and as you finish reading, continue being aware of the rhythm of your breathing. Breathing freely brings vitality to your life, helps it to flow on rather than stay stuck in old patterns. Be on the breath like a bird on the wing.

You don't depend on anyone for air

You can feel so dependent and attached to another person that just the thought of being without them takes your breath away. Sometimes this can be mistaken for love. By liberating your breathing from all restrictive patterns that could have originated as early as birth will help to find your autonomy where you realise that you are not dependent on anyone for your being.

I had an insight quite early on in my practise of Yoga, 'If I realise that I don't depend on anyone for air what is there to confuse me?'

You are not rigidly determined by restrictive breathing patterns set up early on. Breathing is on the threshold of voluntary and involuntary functions, so cultivating awareness of breathing can free you from those repetitive restrictions. To be in control of your breathing makes you realise that you don't depend on anyone for air, or for your essential being. Often people stay in relationships that don't work out of fear of separation anxiety, which could relate to the premature cutting of the umbilical cord, which did take your breath away. Maybe we won't have to stifle each other for fear of letting some breathing space between us. Becoming aware of the relationship between thoughts, feelings and breathing will help you to become more conscious of how often you hold your breath.

Reminds me of Groucho Marx who, while holding a man's pulse, looks at his watch and says, 'Either this man is dead or my watch has stopped.'

If someone next to you is holding their breath notice how it affects your breathing. You'll find yourself holding your breath, too, unless you become conscious of it and able to let go. We tend to overlook how we affect each other on such basic levels. So the more harmonious and in touch we are with our breathing the more harmonious our being and being with each other. *'Conspire'* literally means *'to breathe together.'*

Wait till you can feel the wave of your breath, wait for the spontaneous sigh that comes out of the depths. Ahhhhhh!

Fear of letting go

Once you start to let go you might not like seeing what you've managed so far to suppress. The getting in touch with and being able to acknowledge and accept what we begin to see in ourselves, not just the roses but also the thorns, takes courage. It's not easy to admit to yourself, for instance, that you've been a selfish bitch most of your life. Here's some good news; you don't have to remain a selfish bitch forever if you can manage to own up to it. You might even start seeing the funny side of it. This will release the love rays, which have only been waiting for the opportunity to break through.

The patterns of holding on to a false sense of security, our ideas of who we are, possibly formed in early childhood as ways of 'coping', rather than 'being', run very deep and are tricky to get to. I've discovered how many inhibitions are hiding, among other places, in my vocal chords. The journey to my authentic voice has been a struggle, encountering cobwebs of anger, fear, frustration and hurt that constricted my voice and my soul. What made that journey possible was my voice teacher, Anthea Parashchak, who understands and is not afraid of emotions arising. She encourages, like a good midwife, the deepest energy held in the emotional structures to be released and the real voice to be born. My practice of Yoga and breathing provided the foundation for my voice to begin to open.

Practising Yoga and sharing the fruits of the practice with others is teaching me how to love. I teach what I need to learn. True compassion comes from the heart being in the right place.

Hurt in childhood closes the heart so it doesn't know how to love. Some aboriginal tribes believe that your soul moves away from your body if you have been badly treated as a child. It takes away your confidence, making you focus on your shortcomings instead and stops the flow of life's vitality.

By restoring the flow of the breath we can restore life's vitality and the joy that is our birthright.

Notice your resistance to the full exhalation — *the fear of letting go.*

Acknowledge the fear. Say 'Hello, fear,' and continue breathing. When we let go we have a chance to begin to experience the current of life, the energy force, fearlessness, joyfulness. We can feel the stirrings of the freedom not to deviate from the truth of our being.

The cycles of activity and passivity

The psychological and emotional aspects connected with the full exhalation and full inhalation could be related to the inability to let go and the inability to receive, as well as the fear of emptiness. They also express the cycles of activity and passivity.

At the end of the exhalation the lower abdominal muscles contract to help to expel the air. The more complete the exhalation the more fresh air you will be able to inhale. At the end of the full exhalation the base of the body becomes planted and surrendered to the roots and simultaneously the upper body releases its tensions. Observe and consciously recognise the interconnectedness between surrendering to the ground and releasing upwards as you sit and breathe.

The full exhalation renews your vigour by relaxing the inspiration muscles and allowing new oxygen to enter the blood stream.

Dare to be empty and wait for the wave of the inhalation.

Balance between inhalation and exhalation is related to the balance between the two phases of living: activity and rest.

The most primal ability to give and receive is hidden in your breathing patterns. If your breathing is free your capacity to give and to receive also becomes more open and spontaneous.

A tired body can be re-charged with conscious breathing.

Breathing is happening whether we are aware of it or not. Thoughts and emotions that are suppressed can interfere with the free flow of the breath by maintaining tension in the muscles. Becoming aware of the state of your mind is essential for freeing the breath and letting it find it's natural rhythm.

Restricting breathing is a way of restricting feeling. To breathe freely is to feel.

'It is important for blood balance to breathe deeply. Haemoglobin is one of the important constituents of blood contained in red corpuscles that carry oxygen.'

Sometimes I say this in class because I've read it and it sounds important, but for me, personally, this type of knowledge goes in one ear and out the other without having the least affect on my health. But what does have a profound effect on my well-being is becoming quiet and experiencing the flow of my breath, noticing my attention wander and coming back to my breath over and over again.

We are infused with a *life force* or energy. Inner chatter depletes our energy, and undermines our well-being. You can verify this by your own experience. If you are feeling nervous, stop and become aware of your breathing, you'll realise that it is restricted. We can retain distorted patterns of breathing even after the events that caused the distortion have long passed, like light reaching us from stars long extinguished.

Poor breathing effects our memory and our concentration, so possibly even the natural deterioration of memory could be slowed down with conscious breathing. It is not enough to practise *pranayama*; your awareness of the breath has to extend to everyday activities; to every moment. If you become aware of your breathing, just for a moment you are already participating more fully in the integrated function of body, mind and spirit, in the creative process of life itself.

Step out of the way and allow yourself 'to be breathed'.
Don't hold your breath!
Live on the exhalation.

SIX
Pranayama: breathing exercises

Pranayama means to harmonise the breath and come into relationship with it. To make the respiratory rhythm slow and rhythmical, and to expand the breath.

Before practising pranayama exercises become quiet, listen and acknowledge where you are at this moment. Each one of us has our own unique breathing rhythm that will unfold as restrictive mental and emotional patterns drop away.

Sitting meditation posture

Why is correct posture so important for meditation and breathing?

The spine must be deeply grounded in the base, releasing upwards, allowing the head to balance in line with the spine, so that the subtle forces may flow without hindrance, establishing physical and mental harmony by relaxation and rhythmic breathing. A steady posture and rhythmic breathing creates a state of physical and mental calm that is a good basis for practising meditation.

Sit cross-legged on the edge of a cushion on the floor. If that is not comfortable, sit with your back against a wall. Notice the contact of the sitting bones with the ground. Let the weight distribute evenly onto the sitting bones and let the pelvis become steady and grounded.

Feel the upper body releasing and finding its alignment from the roots, which implies letting go of 'attitudes' in the upper body.

When you feel firm and steady in the base of the spine you will experience the trunk sitting in the pelvis like a good rider on a horse.

Allow an opening across the chest.

Put your hands onto your knees with the palms open, thumbs and index fingers touching, or one hand on top of the other with the thumbs touching.

Tune in to your breathing rhythm.

Do nothing. Don't try to change your breathing rhythm. Just relax and notice the inhalation and exhalation. Let your breathing become harmonious. Let the inhalation flow into exhalation and into inhalation, etc. Slowly allow the exhalation to become deeper.

Follow the exhalation into the lower abdomen till the lower abdomen muscles cave in at the end. Pause. Then let the inhalation come infinitely slowly from the roots, leaving the pelvis firmly grounded.

Let the top of the chest gradually open at the end of the inhalation, without losing the connection to the roots. It is very important to become aware of the top of the chest cavity, which is the narrowest part of the chest and tends to get congested.

Imagine, as you breathe in from the roots the very top of the breastbone lifting at the end of the inhalation.

Breathe in- pause- breathe out- pause - breathe in- pause - breathe out…

Let go of this exercise.

Sit quietly – observing your breath. Observe the sensations accompanying you breathing in the lower abdomen or in the nostrils as the air enters and leaves. Observe thoughts as they arise. Don't follow them, let them go and come back to the sitting and breathing.

Tuning in to your breathing

Sit on the floor in the meditation posture. Close your eyes. Do nothing.

Observe what is on your mind: fear, anxiety, worry, excitement, or just general chatter?

Recognise it,
do nothing.
don't try to change it,
let it be.
Let go of grasping either negative or positive thoughts and emotions, and notice your breathing.
Observe it without changing it.
Listen to your breathing; let it come and go; notice how it begins to get a little deeper all by itself.
Like a deep sigh, which comes unexpectedly from somewhere deep inside, the breath begins to awaken. Follow it without changing it.
Thoughts will arise and intrude.
Recognise the thought as soon as you are able to.
Be present to whatever is going on inside you, without judging, 'oh, here I go again', and when thoughts come up, acknowledge them and continue attending to the breath. It is a very different attitude from approaching the exercise with a forceful wilfulness, that makes breathing exercises part of our ego trip, 'I am good at breathing exercises!'

Initially, becoming conscious of the breath can be a disturbing experience making you aware of how stifled your breath is. When you start releasing your breathing you may come across the same emotional states that made you cut off in the first place. You become aware of how restless the mind is. It may seem that it's all getting worse rather than better. It is important to remember that it's because you are becoming quieter that you are more disturbed by the restlessness, which was there all along.

Each breath is a miracle that leaves plenty of room for wonder and awe, the sense that the breath comes from a source to which we can become attuned and in which we can find solace.

Think of the exhalation as letting go without holding back.

Relax your breathing, do nothing, feel the wave of your breath and then consciously make the exhalation longer. It helps if you make a hissing sound 'sssss' between the teeth to empty the lungs, letting the stream of air synchronise with the sound as you slowly exhale.

At the end of the exhalation, let go, touch the ground wholeheartedly. If the exhalation is complete you will feel the lower abdomen contracting at the end. At the end of the exhalation we get in touch with the centre of gravity below the navel and above the pubic bone.

> Relax the inhalation muscles.
> Don't try to breathe in, don't grasp.
> Wait for the wave of the inhalation.
> Receive the breath like a gift.

Think of the inhalation as receiving without grasping.

It is impossible to over-emphasise the enormous importance of letting the inhalation come from the lower abdomen, with the pelvis deeply grounded after a full exhalation. If you don't breathe from the lower abdomen the upper muscles come into play before the diaphragm has fully expanded. The result is to tense all the muscles of the shoulders, neck and jaw which, in turn, interferes with the circulation around the heart.

The full inhalation opens your chest and rib cage in length, breadth and circumference. In inhalation first the lower abdomen expands, then the stomach, then the chest. If you let your inhalation come infinitely slowly from the lower abdomen it will engage your diaphragm from a deeper place and allow the bottom of your lungs fill with air.

Alternate nostril breathing

> to awaken, balance and harmonise male - female energies,
> to balance the solar and lunar channels in the body,

helps to balance the right and left sides of the body,
has a calming effect on the mind,
helps concentration.

The practice

Put the right thumb on the right nostril,
the ring and the little finger on the left,
the index and the middle finger folded inside.
Close the right nostril, breathe in through the left.
Close the left nostril, breathe out through the right.
Breathe in through the right,
breathe out through the left. etc.
Change nostrils after you have breathed in.

The right hand stays in a precise position the elbow a little up, not sagging so that there is a sense of space and lightness in the whole position of the arm. Practice the above for a few minutes every day.

A spine liberating circular breathing exercise.

Sit on the floor in a cross-legged position.
Feel your sitting bones touching the floor equally, pelvis steady and grounded. Allow your head to find its balance on the broad base of the atlas.
This will give you a sense of freedom in the neck muscles.

Imagine a point above the crown of your head.
Imagine breathing in from that point in a circle going around your body and ending at the base of the spine.
Imagine the exhalation starting from the base of the spine and going upwards beyond the crown of the head.
In a muscular way the exhalation goes down to the base of the spine but your awareness goes with the upward movement of the spine.
So it is a two- way movement, like two lifts moving in opposite directions.

The effect of this exercise is to enable the spine to become grounded, releasing upwards, freeing the spinal column.

You can also do this exercise lying down.
Lie on the floor with your knees bent, feet slightly apart about the width of your hips, heels slightly wider than the toes. This helps to broaden the lower back.
Relax and tune in to your breathing rhythm.
Gradually make the exhalation longer.
Feel how, in a muscular way, the full exhalation goes down to the root of the
spine at the same time as it goes upwards, freeing the spine upwards.
As you breathe out imagine again the two lifts going in opposite directions. As one reaches the bottom of the spine, the other goes up beyond the crown of your head.

Kumbaka - breath retention

Breathe in to the count of 5.
Hold the breath to the count of 15 without tensing up.
Exhale to the count of 10.
The basic ratio of this exercise is 1:3:2 – so you can change it according to your needs making it longer or shorter.

Repeat this cycle five times.

Imagine, as you are sitting with the pelvis as steady as a mountain, the lungs
like the branches and leaves of a tree, receiving nourishment through the roots.

This exercise is empowering and energising. It helps to expand the lungs and to focus the mind on the breath.

Kapalabati - Scull cleanser

A cleansing exercise that helps to get grounded and clear the head, strengthen the centre of gravity, release the upper body, free the neck and allow the head to balance naturally.

Quick short exhalations contracting the muscle below the navel
To start with do 20 quick exhalations keeping a steady beat in the lower abdomen. Stay in tune with your inner rhythm.
Repeat the cycle 3 times.
At the end of the 20th exhalation, pause, let the inhalation come.
Relax.

Counting the breath

Count to five as you breathe in,
pause at the end of the inhalation,
count to five as you breathe out,
pause at the end of the exhalation.

After practising a breathing exercise, it's very profound to be able to let go of the exercise, allowing the breath to do what it wants to do to flow freely.

For women

Breathe into your breasts, scanning the breasts with your awareness and releasing all the stagnant energy. Breathe into your nipples.

Breathing awareness during activities.

When you are walking feel your feet touching the ground and the upper body releasing infinitely to the sky. Synchronise the breath with your steps. Becoming aware of breathing during all your activities will improve the concentration and co-ordination in your sitting, standing, walking, running, dancing, working, etc.

It will help the spine to find it's natural position and release upwards.

***Pranayama exercises help us to become conscious
and expand the breath
but the most essential thing
is to stay in touch with your breathing
and be at ease with your breath.***

SEVEN
More Yoga Stories

It's hard to say!

T. arrives for a Yoga lesson and says he is tired.

I suggest, 'Lie on your back with knees bent, feet in line with the hips and just feel the contact the back is making with the floor. Relax. Let gravity do the work.'

He says, 'I might appear not very relaxed to you but compared with some people I *am* relaxed, I don't feel tense.'

'It's all relative', I say.

We do a few simple postures.

I can see the muscles at the back of his legs like tight ropes; his shoulders pulled up to his ears, his lower back weak and pulled up, his feet not grounded.

Lying down to relax at the end of the session he huffs and puffs and says, 'I can't relax'.

'Do you feel less tired than when you arrived?'

'It's hard to say', he says, pulling his sweater over his face.

After a pause he says, 'I'm feeling angry,' hastily adding, 'and I don't know why'.

'Do you know who you are angry with?'

'I don't know. It's hard to say.'

I say, 'When you let go of tensions, feelings emerge that have been held in the tight muscles.'

He says, 'I might appear tense to you, but I am very relaxed in comparison with some people.'

'Where is it supposed to hurt?'

'We shouldn't ask why we are wounded, only that our wounds should be healed.'

F. sits on the floor with both legs stretched in front, in a Yoga posture called *Parshchimotanasana*.
(I notice that my life hasn't changed much from knowing the Sanskrit names of the postures, but I *have* found out a lot about my attitudes from forward bends. To bend forward with an attitude of trying to reach the goal, which in this case is the feet, is doing what a Zen master said so aptly, *'losing the roots and reaching out for the tree tops, or pulling at the stalks to make the wheat grow faster.'*)

I say, 'Feel your sitting bones on the ground. Let your weight go evenly into your sitting bones, relax your breath, exhale and make a feeling contact with the ground. Notice how your upper body responds naturally by releasing as you plant the roots deeper.

Let gravity do the job; let the backs of your legs release to the ground. *Feel* the contact. Whatever you are doing do less, you'll find your legs will get closer to the ground if you make a *feeling* contact.

Let your hip joints release towards the ground. Once you have established the connection to the ground, the spine begins to want to lengthen. Notice if your knees begin to lift up. Come back, breathe your knees down, keep planting the roots.

Moving forward is growing from the roots. It's a matter of breathing and waiting for the hamstring muscles to lengthen and become flexible enough to allow the spine to elongate forward.

The forward movement is like a tree growing from the roots, with the leaves and branches infinitely open to the sky.'

F. asks, 'Is it supposed to hurt here?' pointing to her left hip.

I'm often asked, *'Is this where it's supposed to hurt?'* I feel that this question touches on being disconnected from our own authority. Get in touch with your own experience. Tune into your body and stay with what is there attentively. You can release tension by breathing and attending to *your* unique experience of each posture.

The posture is the map, not the territory. The territory is your unique experience of it. Pain is a way of drawing your attention to blocked energy. It's not that *pain is good for you,* but often we only start paying attention when it hurts.

All concepts of how things *ought to be* have to be dropped in order to experience the body directly.

'I have pain in my hip, don't know why?'

This reminds me of the Buddhist story about the guy who got shot by an arrow and, when a friend wanted to take the arrow out, said, 'No, don't take it out, I first want to know who sent it and what material it is made of.'

His friend replied, 'Let's get it out first and then see what it's made of.'

I feel it is not helpful to think 'why is this pain there'; in fact it stands in the way of breathing and letting go. After you've let go then the insight of what it was all about might emerge.

Well adjusted to crooked ways

'Lie on your back, with your knees bent, feet parallel and in line with your hips.'

I look at A. Her pelvis is out of line with her shoulders, her head is to one side and her whole body looks like a zigzag. I put her head straight, asking her to bring her pelvis in line with her shoulders and feet.

She lies still for a while and then says, 'I feel crooked.'

I suggest that she *look* at her body. She looks and says she can see that she is straight but she still *feels* crooked.

If it looks straight but feels crooked it could be that we've become well adjusted to crooked ways. It takes attentiveness and a lot of patience to allow the body to unfold to its natural alignment and for the inner awareness to align to the newly aligned body.

How are you?

'Oh, mustn't grumble.'
'Fair to middling.'
'Bearing up.'
'So-so.'
'Fantastic!'
'Surviving.'
'Can't complain.'
'Not so bad.'
'Plodding on.'
'Could be worse.'
'Oh, all right, looking forward to going away.'

Proprioceptive awareness

B. says his legs hurt.

I suggest, 'Lie on your back and we'll do the leg-stretching exercises.'

After a while I notice that his hips look more open, his legs more relaxed.

'How do your legs feel now?' He starts feeling them with his hands.

I say, 'What I mean is - how does it feel from inside? Proprioceptive awareness, you know?'

'I know, I know!'

'So, how does it feel?'

'I don't know, you tell me.'

'Did you notice my restlessness?'

K. is lying on the floor with a bolster under his knees, which is helpful for taking the weight off his legs and hips, allowing the pelvis to relax and the spine to align.

I say, 'Do nothing. Let the weight of your body sink to the floor. Acknowledge what's on your mind, give yourself a lot of space with all your thoughts and feelings Don't try to change them, relax with them, accept yourself, and feel how your breathing becomes deeper all by itself.'

He lies for a few seconds and his hand suddenly shoots towards his nose and gives it a scratch. After a few more moments his hand suddenly, jerkily scratches his chin.

I say, 'Try this exercise. Notice the impulse to scratch your face and stop for a moment before acting on it, and then scratch it if you have to.'

He lies still for a moment and suddenly his hand moves again to his chin, and he scratches it.

He opens his eyes and smiles; 'I had to.'

I say, 'This exercise will help you to become aware of your restlessness and relax.'

K. smiles his disarming smile and says, 'Did you notice restlessness?'

'If you stay mindful of sensations, thoughts, feelings, attending to them and doing nothing, then you can go through thresholds of pain, irritability, fear and restlessness and transform them into peacefulness. But first of all become aware that you are indeed restless.'

'Should we be mindful of our feet while brushing our teeth?'

'Can't do any harm. Say 'hello' to the earth and make wholehearted contact with it as soon as you stand up on your feet every morning, or whenever you can remember. Notice how it helps your spine release upward, which is its natural movement. We don't need to hold the upper body if we connect to the feet and the upward movement.'

'I pulled a muscle, should I come?' (A phone call before a class.)

'Yes, why not? You can relax, breathe and align your body. If emotional reactions come up and you start feeling frustrated that you can't do what others are doing, it's a good opportunity to practise letting go, being present, starting from where you are at this moment and not where you'd like to be. It will give your body the opportunity to relax and the pulled muscle will heal quicker.'

Death Pose

'How long should I stay in the death pose?'

When you start snoring and wake yourself up it's probably time to stop! On a more serious note, the death pose is the hardest of all poses. It requires total surrender of the body and an alert, awake awareness. This is the goal of the death pose.

What happens in the beginning is that most people fall asleep, because relaxation is commonly associated with falling asleep. It takes time and practice to be able to stay totally quiet and still and yet exquisitely aware. We do the death pose for as long as it takes to arrive at the stillness of the body and mind without falling asleep. But if you do fall asleep enjoy it and hopefully feel refreshed.

Using what ever comes up to grow towards living in the present

F: I've found the experience of Yoga with you so different from all the other teachers I have had. You talk about *using whatever comes up to grow towards being able to live in the present, by going through it and getting to know it rather than avoiding and repressing it*. To me that's the difference – you allow that we've only got what we've got, dark, ugly as it may seem, that's all we've got to work with.

Mina: Yes, it's true; it's vital to connect bodily posture with thoughts, emotions and breathing.

F: I don't believe that people tie up enough the connection between the psyche and the body. But you talk about it all the time in class, that psychological blocks are locked and stored in the body and by becoming aware of and releasing the tensions we can become aware of what's hiding there and eventually free ourselves by letting go.

For instance, when you told me that you had been living in your neck all your pre-Yoga life, it made me aware that so had I. At first I found it hard to make that connection, but now I can feel where these blocks are. And that they are not only physical.

All that history stuck in my neck makes it impossible to have clarity about what's really going on in the present moment.

The moment you slow down and say hello to the present moment,
meaning and vitality are here to greet you.

EIGHT

Yoga by e-mail:
Trikonasana – the controversial Triangle Pose

*T*he Triangle pose, in Sanskrit, *Trikonasana*, needs and deserves a lot of attention.

I received the following email from a friend in Jerusalem who has practised Yoga for many years.

The subject of this email was *'hip-hop'!*
Did lots of Yoga in Greece and realised I need a teacher to show me what's happening to my hip when I do Trikonasana - the sideways bend, plus other bits and pieces.

I replied:
What comes to mind about your hip is this: before you bend to the side or forward, lift the knee caps up into your hips deeply, distinctly and evenly, so the hips feel steady. And observe the difference.

She came back:
I can't bend to the side, it starts hurting

I replied:
OK, one more thing comes to mind as I read what you are saying.

1. *Put your feet in the triangle position.*
2. *Stand, connect to your feet, breathe into them, do nothing. Stay in that position and feel the weight going into the centre of the heels. Let your toes stretch. Let the energy flow beyond the tips of the toes. Get in touch with the axis of the spine from the base of the spine to the crown of the head.*
3. *If you are bending to the right put your left hand on the sacrum and guide it towards the tail. Keep guiding it. Lift the right kneecap towards the hip. Establish a firm connection there and keep the sacrum lengthening. This is your focus - lengthening the sacrum and keeping the right hip steady, so the right thigh is rotating outwards. Now you've got a steady triangle.*
4. *Then bring the right shoulder forward, left shoulder back, opening the chest without letting the right hip move forward. That will help to keep your neck free so the head will naturally want to turn towards the ceiling. Steady feet, steady hips, sacrum lengthening and chest opening without changing the triangle.*

She replied:
Thanks Mina, you feel so present. As I follow your advice it makes me smile. I'll let you know after I've tried it for a while. It seems quite a deep change has happened and is important to attend to.

A week later:
You are a genius and I don't say it lightly - that works like magic, all is smooth and my hips' panic attack eased, comforted, cured, and reassured by following your advice exactly.

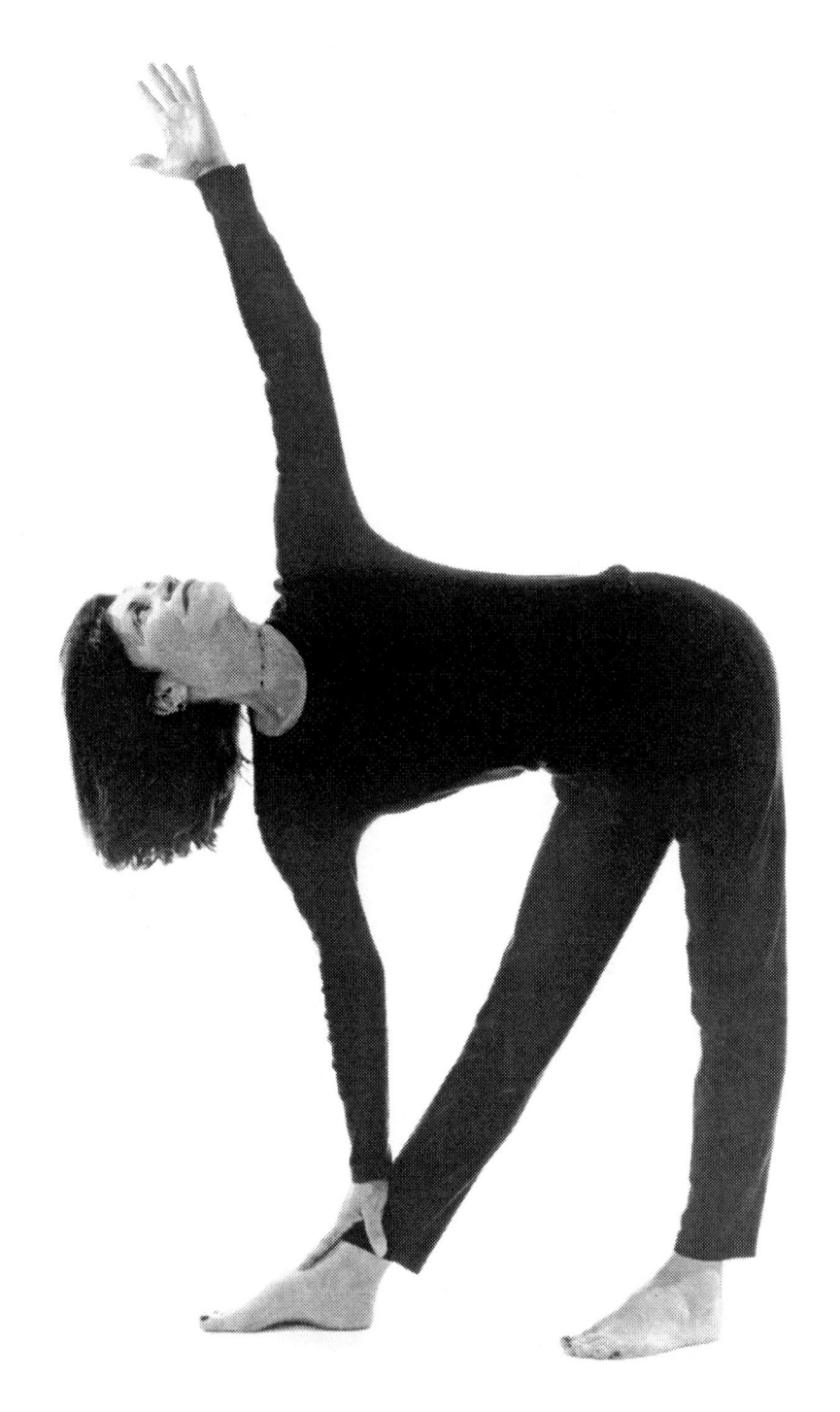

Trikonasana

NINE

All the things you can do lying on your back ...and improve your health

We cannot release that of which we are not aware.

The body is a storehouse of early memories, often traumatic, which can contribute to many ailments if not released. But in order to release them we first need to become aware of them. We cannot release that of which we are not aware. Practising Yoga postures mindfully can be a way to get to know and release these troublesome old tensions, helping us get in touch with the inherent unity of mind, body, spirit.

If you concentrate your attention on your body with *feeling*, screening it with awareness, expect a lot of emotional steam to rise as the tensions, which have been hiding in the tight muscles, are being released. On the way back to yourself you might encounter the same emotions of fear and hurt that made you disconnect in the first place.

The choice is either to ignore these painful emotions, concentrating on being 'good' at 'doing' the posture, or to acknowledge them, coming 'out of the closet' and into closer contact with yourself. By having the courage to make this *feeling* connection you begin to awaken the body's natural intelligence.

When the body is out of balance it goes against the life force, which can make us feel as if life is against us.

When the body is balanced it functions effortlessly. A new body image begins to surface in our consciousness, free from all the conditioned images. When we accept our body our immune system gets stronger and our inner beauty has a chance to shine forth. Lucky for us there is such a thing as inner beauty since the outer beauty gets a bit ragged at the edges, let's face it!

Conscious lying down

> Lie down on your back. Bend your knees, your feet on the floor the width of your hips apart, with the heels slightly wider than the toes. This gives your lower back a chance to broaden and open.
> Take your head in your hands and elongate the back of your neck. Hold your head for a few minutes with your chin coming towards your chest and let the tension escape from the base of your skull.
> Then put your head down mindfully in line with your spine. Be aware of your neck being the continuation of the spine and not just this little thing sticking out and stiffening up at the slightest provocation.
> Place your arms by your sides, slightly away from your body, so they don't cling to the body, giving your lymphatic glands room to breathe. If you're not sure if you are straight, take a good look, and imagine that if your nose grew like Pinocchio's it would come between your knees.

Give yourself a big hug.

> Get hold of your shoulder blades and open the space between them. Give a
> little wriggle and let that space open more.
> Feel the connection between this space and the space around your heart. We don't need to *try* and open the space around the heart. If we travel down the spine with our exhalation and let the base of the spine become grounded the space around the heart will open as a consequence, like a flower.

Do nothing.
Acknowledge your internal weather, thoughts, feelings and physical sensations.
Give yourself space to be with everything that is going on inside.
Notice, after a while, that as you open to and accept your inner world, your breathing begins to relax all by itself.
Stay with it, connecting with your breathing rhythm and wait till you are at ease with your breath.

Wait for the wave of the breath to come, like a spontaneous deep sigh.

As you tune into your breathing rhythm gradually make the exhalation longer. Exhale on the sound 'sssss'.
At the end of the exhalation feel your lower abdomen cave in, pause, touch the ground wholeheartedly and receive the inhalation.
Pause at the end of the inhalation and again exhale on the sound 'sssss'.
Relax the breath. Don't push, let the sound and the stream of air synchronise, so that the exhalation on the sound 'sssss' is not mechanical.
At the end of the exhalation feel your lower abdomen cave in.
Pause and let the inhalation come.

Become aware of the alignment of your body.

Awareness of our body alignment and symmetry should be at least as much a part of our hygiene as washing and deodorising ourselves.

Lie on the floor with your knees bent, feet slightly apart. Let your back release to the floor. Enjoy the contact. Feel the sacrum in the centre. The sacrum, the sacred bone, is fused from the waist down to the tailbone. Feel it, become familiar with it. It is the base of the spine and if it's in the centre it provides a good foundation for the spine to release and lengthen upwards.

Feel the interconnectedness of the whole spine. Freedom in you neck is directly connected to being grounded in the base of the spine.

Whatever you are doing do less.

Take your arms up in the air lazily, making a feeling connection with your wrists, elbows and shoulders. Feel the energy flowing through your arms.
Cross your arms over each other the other way, the non-habitual way.
Repeat the same exercise, breathing out on the sound 'sssss'.
Take your arms and legs up in the air like a beetle lying upside down.
Feel all the joints of the limbs relaxing. Let your joints be playful. Hug your knees gently.
Meditate on the thought 'holding without holding on'.

Notice a wave of release going through your body as you let go of all unnecessary holding.

Doing this exercise only, every day, will make your body more supple, your breathing freer, and most of all, help you to establish a feeling connection to your body.

Energy is never static, it is in a constant state of movement but we can get stuck and become rigid. Practising the following asanas with awareness helps to get the breath to flow, releasing blocked energy. They will connect you to your body, to your breath, to gravity and the release that comes from it.

Twists

Spinal twists stimulate circulation in the abdomen and abdominal muscles. Twists have a beneficial effect on the flexibility of the spine. The action of rotation and de-rotation improves the condition of the soft tissue discs by allowing them to absorb fresh nutrients and get rid of wastes. This stops the discs from dehydrating and degenerating, which is often responsible for shrinking height, as we get older.

Gentle twist to release the spine.

Hold underneath your knees and take them to the left.
While still holding under your knees straighten the legs from the calves to the heels. Bend the knees and put your left hand on top of the knees.
Be economical with your movement. Simply take your hand from under your knees and place it on top of the knees.

Leg stretches.

Lie on your back, hugging your knees.
Hold gently without pulling into your shoulders keeping your neck relaxed and
your shoulders relaxed and 'shruggable.'
Stretch your right leg on the floor.
Become aware of your pelvis being in the centre. If you are not sure where the centre is, tilt a little to the left, a little to the right, and come back to the centre.
Put a belt around your right foot and stretch the leg up. Breathe into your right
hip, let it release towards the ground, lift the kneecap towards the hip and stretch the leg from the calf to the heel.
Now take the right leg to the side. Hold this position.
Rest your leg on a cushion if the stretch is too strenuous.
Bring the leg back to the centre.
Breathe into the right hip, elongate from the hip towards the waist and take
the leg across.
If the left shoulder is very tight bring the arm across as well and breathe out into the feet, as if you are standing on them, and with the next long exhalation turn to the left and bring you arm across as smoothly as possible.

Relaxing and centering the eyes

These life's windows on the soul
Distort the heavens from pole to pole
And lead us to believe a lie
That we see 'with' not 'through' the eye.
William Blake

An exercise to relax the eyes

Lie on your back with knees bent and feet slightly apart, about the width of your hips.
Lengthen the back of your neck, open the space between the shoulder blades and relax the arms by the sides slightly away from the body, so that the arms are not clinging to the body and there is space in the armpits.
Acknowledge the thoughts, or the emotional weather inside, recognise, accept, let it be and let your attention settle on the eyes. You might become aware of how jumpy and restless they are, and how the muscles around the eyes tense.
Exhale deeply, allow the muscles around the eyes to relax, let your eyes sink to the bottom of the eye sockets, wait for them to reach to the bottom.
Imagine them like two pebbles sinking into a lake till they reach the bottom. Feel your eyes becoming still. Direct your gaze slightly down without straining. Exhale, touch the ground whole-heartedly and let all your muscles empty of tension. Feel the sensations of the body touching the ground. Don't **try** to breathe in, let the your inhalation come all by itself. Allow your chest to open.
Feel your eyes quiet and serene like the eyes of the Buddha.

TEN

Hips are for Swinging, Shoulders are for Shrugging

Forget everything you've ever been told about what it means to 'stand on your own two feet' and find your own connection to Mother Earth.

Finding your feet.

I remember the days when standing meant shifting from one foot to the other, shoulders aching, neck stiff, not feeling at home in my skin. Awareness of how we place our feet, or the lack of it, affects our whole body. If our feet are fully open and balanced, making good contact with the ground, our body will naturally feel free with the spine elongating upwards as we walk or stand. The way we place our feet helps to free the knees, and to broaden and strengthen the lower back. Deepening the connection of the soles of the feet with the ground also helps the circulation of blood to the heart.

It is high up on the evolutionary scale to have our feet firmly on the ground and to let our bodies release upwards.

Human beings stood up on two feet. The debate is still going on about what this means. Having our feet on the ground certainly doesn't mean being mundane and boring and forgetting our dreams. Anyone with even a drop of Gypsy in their soul will know that giving up on our dreams just won't do.

'They' told us, *Stand on your own two feet,* but omitted to tell us that if we did we'd experience tremendous freedom in our whole being, we wouldn't be all top-heavy with no foundation.

Standing on our feet doesn't mean being grounded in the sense of *be practical and put those nonsense dreams out of your head.* But it does require being fully awake to have your feet on the ground and your head in the sky.

'I hate my feet!' says a woman in my Yoga class. This in response to an exercise we are doing, sitting on the heels with ankles together. Since it is difficult to keep the ankles aligned we use a belt around the top of the heels to bring the ankles into alignment. When I bring her attention to her ankles being too far apart she says,

'It's because I have disgusting feet.'

This made me wonder how many negative images are imprinted in our minds that interfere with our direct perception of the body as it really is.

I wonder how much of life is wasted on worrying about, 'I am too tall, too thin, too fat, too short. My lips are too thin and my breasts are too big, I should have them diminished. My breasts are too small, I should have them enlarged; I need a face-lift, etc. etc.'

Acknowledging and releasing negative images is part of the process of becoming whole.

Standing can become relaxing and interesting.

We'd never be bored, and our muscle tone would remain alive and 'interested', even in a simple standing position, if we'd stay in touch with the vitality needed for the constant rediscovery of our balance. Rediscovering and securing a well-integrated position while standing frees the muscles of their old habits.

A baby learning to stand enjoys an exciting game of losing and finding his/her balance. Later we take it for granted, and lose the vitality, which comes from necessity for constant renewal.

'I have flat feet'

Flat feet, where the inner arch of the foot has dropped, is not a *fait accompli*, it is a bad habit that has been around for a very long time.

'Ah but my mother also has flat feet'

She has also had this habit for a long time. People say it runs in the family. Sure it runs because nobody will stop and consider whether it has to run. If you stop, place your feet, have a good look and use your common sense your inner and outer ankle-bones should be aligned. If you keep dropping your inner ankle-bones for a few generations, yes, it will run …and run …and run in the family.

Feet stretching exercise

> Stand with your feet parallel, heels slightly wider than the toes.
> Hold one wrist behind your back; let your shoulders relax.
> Bend your right knee and let your weight go into your left foot.
> Feel your right leg empty.
> Lift your right heel up and stretch your foot from the centre of the ball of the foot and then place the heel down again.
> Lift the toes and stretch them so the foot becomes longer and wider.
> Spread the toes.
> Repeat the same on the other side.
> Notice how your neck tends to get involved.
> It's quite an art to let it stay quiet.
> Stand, letting the weight go evenly into both feet.
> Close your eyes, do nothing, let go of thoughts and connect up to your breathing.

Three way feet exercise

1. Sit on your heels, breathe your weight down into your sitting bones and release your pelvis.
2. Turn onto your toes, knees down. If this is uncomfortable keep your hands on the floor to release the pressure.
3. Squatting, drop your head, breathe and relax. You could put a cushion under your heels to bring them down. Be as comfortable as you possibly can.
   Repeat the sequence a few times, with awareness of your breathing.

Effects

Opens the soles of the feet.
Makes the ankles flexible.
Stretches the Achilles tendons.
Opens the arches of the feet.
Opens the hips.
Improves circulation, digestion, respiration, and heart condition.

Standing with 100% enthusiasm in your feet ...or 10% will do!

Place your feet parallel, about a foot apart, heels a little wider than your toes. Give yourself time and space to truly experience standing on your own two feet.

Close your eyes, feel the contact your feet are making with the ground.

Relax your breathing; let go of tension.

Feel your weight going down into your heels and experience the upward movement which comes from surrender to the ground.

The heel is the biggest bone in the foot, so the weight naturally goes down into the heels, if we let it.

'But I feel as if I am falling backwards!'

The Distracted Centipede – a Yoga Experie

'That's why, thank God, you have toes. Use them!'

Feel the base of the toes making contact with the ground.

Let your toes be free and the energy flow beyond the tips of the toes.

As you stand, feel gravity pulling your feet down.

Plant the base of your big toe firmly and imagine a line going from the base of your big toe diagonally across to the outside of your heel.

Let it go all round your heel and then diagonally across to the base of your little toe.

Spread your toes, so there is distance between each toe.

Feel the sensations in the soles of your feet as they touch the ground.

Feel your anklebones, the inner and the outer in the centre and your feet dropping away from the anklebones.

Let your feet become quiet and grounded without your legs getting rigid.

For your body to experience an upward release your feet have to make a deep connection with the ground.

Feel the outside of your knees opening.

A question that is often asked is, 'Should I lock my knees?'

'No, lock is not the word. The knees don't only open backwards but also laterally from side to side. Imagine the back of the knees grinning! It takes time and practise to get in touch with that lateral movement, so don't worry if you don't feel it yet, it will come.'

Centre your pelvis. Don't push the front bones of your pelvis forward as this unbalances the natural curves of your spine.

The spine works in two ways: the sacrum moves towards the ground like a dinosaur's tail, and, from the small of the back, releases upward toward the sky.

The energy in the area around the spot under the bra strap in the dorsal spine tends to get blocked and stagnant, and needs special attention.

I said to a couple in a Yoga class, 'Let the spot under the bra strap liven up and release upwards, women know it from first hand experience, men, from second hand experience.'

The man said, 'Don't talk to me about bra straps, it will put me off Yoga.'

'Aha! That is the crux of the matter, bring Yoga into bra straps!'

Experience the joy of standing on your own two feet.

Imagine yourself like a snake charmer charming your spine out of its base.

Stay with your inner rhythm; attend to your own individual experience of it.

And don't get beside yourself with Yoga! If you follow the instructions too literally, you'll be missing out on your own experience.

Perky Navel

Whether you are sitting, standing or walking, become aware of your navel; how it tends to collapse in a despondent sort of way! Become aware of your pubic bone in the centre and feel as if your navel is gradually growing from the pubic bone. That secure support at the base creates the upward releasing movement of the spine consequently opening the narrowest top chest cavity.

The head

The head is the theatre of the soul.
Cecil Collins – artist

The head should be up there in a dignified fashion, balanced on top of the atlas, the uppermost cervical vertebra supporting the skull. If the head is centred and balanced on the broad base of the atlas, it will not put any strain on the neck. For the head to be balanced with the neck releasing, the body must be centred at the base of the spine. When the neck is stiff it is a sign that we are pulled up into the head.

To free the neck and allow the head to balance we need to let go of the attitudes we are clinging to in the upper body and surrender to the ground. A head that is held habitually off centre, to one side, or thrown back, creates tension in the muscles holding it off balance. Allowing the spine to find its axis from the root will bring the neck into its natural alignment. The head balances easily on its support when the main structure of the whole body is in balance.

If all of us humans on this planet would stand from the feet upward, and think of the head as the last to come in line with the spine, like a flower on top of the stem, the world would become a friendlier place!

Have mercy on the base of your skull!

This is where the spinal chord and the brain meet, so it makes sense to keep it free and flowing.

Make tiny little nodding movements like a Mandarin doll, backwards and forwards and side to side, the smaller the movement the deeper the feeling connection.

Become aware of the freedom in your neck.

Imagine your neck starting from the root of your spine.

Free the base of your scull.

Let your head gently release upwards and balance effortlessly on top of the Atlas.

This will align your head with the axis of your spine.

The base of the skull, where a lot of tension accumulates and where obstinacy sits, is where the spinal cord reaches the brain …have mercy on it! Let go of this tension, and allow freedom of circulation, so that the natural cranial rhythm is restored.

The puzzled neck

The neck is a busybody; it will get involved in every movement if you let it. If you pay attention you'll notice that your neck is busy all the time. The way to release your neck is to connect to the root of your spine and experience the neck as continuation of the spine.

If the head is off centre the weight on the neck will be heavy. Rock your head like a delicately balanced weight and feel it becoming lighter. Then the neck will find its true alignment and support from the base.

Shoulders are for shrugging

'Shoulders are from God – and burdens too.'
Anonymous

There is a common misconception that shoulders are for carrying burdens and heavy responsibility. That is the case if you are not in touch with your centre of gravity, the source of authentic power. Shoulders are for shrugging. They should be free and loose if you live and move from your centre. Let your shoulders drop onto your shoulder girdle. Let them come home.

The sternum – breast- bone

While standing try to push your rib cage forward, noticing how the lower end of the sternum gets pushed forward and how this compresses the top part of the chest and unbalances the spinal curves. One of the physical expressions of depression is the top part of the chest being compressed. The upper chest cavity must be deep to ensure the best functioning of the upper parts of the lungs and heart. Become aware of keeping the rib cage connected to the spine and not pushed forward. When balance is restored the connection to our vital energy is restored.

Stretching the arms up

Stand consciously.

Swing your arms like pendulums from your shoulder joints, with awareness of the centre of your heels grounded and stable.
Gradually let your arms swing higher, letting them fly up without pulling up into your shoulders.
Don't pull yourself up with your roots.
Don't lose your roots when the wind comes and blows your branches.

Hold one wrist and stretch, feeling the stretch between the heel and the wrist,
like the two ends of a piece of elastic, your hipbones staying steady. Repeat on the other side.
Then link hands and stretch both arms. Then link your hands in the un-habitual way, the other thumb and index finger in front, and stretch again.
Release the arms loosely and drop them making the sound - Ha! - from the centre of your being, expressing in that sound *everything you ever wanted to say and didn't know how to.*

Standing and dropping forward.

Stand with your feet about a foot apart, heels a little wider than the toes.
Feel the contact your feet are making with the ground.
Feel your kneecaps lifting into your hip joints, deeply, distinctly and evenly.
Drop forward, allowing your spine to release from the root.
Let your neck release.
Breathe out on the sound 'Ah' till you feel your lower abdomen cave in.
Then breathe in from the lower abdomen.
Repeat a few times.

Plant your feet again and slowly come up as if growing from your feet.

As you come up notice if you are involving your neck.
Stop, release your neck and continue growing from your feet.
Feel your weight going into the centre of your heels.
Come back to the centre.
Get in touch with the axis of your spine.
Feel your neck lengthening and the head balancing lightly on top of the atlas.
Feel the outer contours of your whole body expanding your energy field.

Doing only this exercise just a few times can free your upper body and make you feel refreshed.

Hips are for swinging

Let your hips swing!

Watch a dog walking and see how he swings his hips. He's not trying to be provocative; swinging the hips is nature's way of ensuring a release of the spine.

Swing your hips! Wag your tail! Free the energy of all the cobwebs. Let there be wildness in your hips! You can have wild hips and a faithful heart.

When walking uphill, you'll find you expend much less effort if you let your hips swing. Notice the inhibition sitting in your hips that doesn't allow them to swing freely. Profound emotional release and liberation can happen as a consequence of the hips opening.

Conscious walking

Becoming conscious of how you stand, sit, walk, lie down and breathe will make your body much more supple. The state of complete bodily relaxation has its roots, physically, in the feet. When you walk, don't 'put the cart before the horse', in other words don't lead with your chin, let your legs do the walking.

How much lighter your body feels if your legs carry it rather than your upper body dragging your legs along! All too often we see people walking with their chins up, leaving their pelvis behind.

When you are walking:
Become aware of your feet and feel them contacting the ground.
Relax your breath, stay in touch with your rhythm.
Let your shoulders relax and come home onto your shoulder girdle.
Allow your neck to elongate out of its base and your head to elevate upwards.
Move from your hips with your upper body releasing.
As your feet touch the ground a wave arises from gravity, elongating the spine as you move.

Walking slowly and mindfully doesn't have to feel or look weird and creepy. I once met a meditation master on a silent retreat in the south of Thailand. We got up at 4.30 a.m., had a 'shower' by ladling water from large cisterns outside over our bodies. Although women and men stayed in different parts of the meditation centre we still had to wear sarongs while we showered, for modesty.

We then walked half an hour to the house of the Master, to listen to the *Dharma* talk in his garden. He was 89, sitting in full lotus position, giving his talk while chickens strutted about with their chicks, cats nursed their kittens, dogs sniffed about for food, birds sang and flowers opened. From time to time, a rooster would alight on his shoulder. He just continued talking about mindfulness. His instruction for our walk back was, 'Walk without a walker.'

**By making closer contact with the ground
you begin to experience the upward movement of the spine
and you realise that there is no need to hold on.**

*Dharma – truth, law, norm, refers to the teachings of the Buddha

ELEVEN

Yoga and Sex

'Once realisation is accepted that even between the closest human beings infinite distance continues to exist, a wonderful living side-by-side can grow up if they succeed in loving the distance between them that makes it possible to see the other whole against a wide sky.'
Rainer Maria Rilke

High heels, orgasm, tightness in the pelvis etc.

You wouldn't expect to find Bruce Forsythe appearing in a Yoga book but I've found the following question and answer in his show 'Play your cards right' significant.

The question: If 'the wife' woke up in an amorous mood on a Monday morning, how many men out of a hundred said they would worry about being late for work?

One contestant answered enthusiastically, 'Oh, I wouldn't. You take what you get.'

It seems the cliché *men take ...women give* is still alive and thriving in our minds and bodies. We will remain confused about what it means to be a man or a woman, and what give and take is really all about, as long as we continue to take our cues from current fashions or traditions, rather than refreshing our way of being with each other from our own experiences.

This guy dies and goes to heaven. Up in heaven he sees two signs. One sign says, 'real men', and there is one man standing next to it. The other sign says, 'hen pecked men' and there is a long queue. The guy is not quite sure where to go so he asks the guy in the 'real men' queue why he is standing there.

He says, 'Oh, my wife told me to.'

That's another common image imprinted in our minds.

What does it mean to be an adult?

From experience I am learning that becoming adult means getting in touch with love in myself, forgiving and letting go of the resentment of not getting it, or not getting it the way I wanted it. Then *loving* becomes an active part of my life rather than a passive waiting *to be loved* in a chronic Sleeping Beauty state.

If we can get to know and relax with our own feelings we'll have the inner space to let each other be. If we are not able to be open and present to our own feelings and sensations we won't be able to be present to the intensity of feelings in sexual union.

In the movies I grew up with, sexual intercourse showed the lovers mauling each other for a few minutes and then frantically galloping towards orgasm. This was supposed to be passion. How can you enjoy and appreciate the scenery from a speeding train? The alternative was Greta Garbo and Robert Taylor whose mere gazing into each other's eyes sent *frissons* up my spine but they looked as if they never did 'it' at all!

No wonder we experience melancholy and post-orgasmic depression, if sex is the only transcendent experience that lifts us out of our everyday life and gives us a momentary break from the torments of our busy minds and bodies.

The fear of opening out after we've been severely hurt can make us contract physically and emotionally. If we don't address this contracted state and develop ways of allowing the energy to flow, we might be holding on to concepts and staying out of touch with our immediate experience. Getting to know your feelings and mastering the flow of the breath will lead to more relaxation and abandonment to your deep inner rhythms, so that sexual intimacy will give birth to joy, not melancholy.

A friend told me he read an article in the newspaper quoting a chiropractor, who claimed that high heels are not good for women, because they distort the posture and cause undue tension and pressure in the pelvis. He linked it to women having difficulties with orgasm because they are so tight in the pelvis from wearing high heels!

I think tightness comes from deep inhibition that hasn't become conscious and hasn't been released. Loose dresses and sandals and apparent openness don't necessarily mean true openness. It's surprising how many women can't have orgasms. The chiropractor said that high heels tend to deaden the feeling in the pelvis. Ok, if a woman has a shortened, pulled up sacrum and pain in the lower back I wouldn't advocate that she wear high heels. But I wouldn't focus on that as the substitute for becoming conscious and working on opening emotionally and physically to what is really going on in her body, mind and heart.

Swinging the hips is associated with being loose and promiscuous. Even in our 'free' age the hips of the western man and woman are still laden with memories of inhibition. Get your grannies out of every nook and cranny!

Vaginal orgasm! Why, what else? To settle for that little twitch-twitch in the clitoris that dilutes all the real erotic feelings by bringing them too quickly to the surface, not allowing them to rise on their own accord from the mystical depths? Men stimulate the clitoris to prepare women to 'come' because they are anxious that they won't last long enough for her to have a real orgasm. Maybe it's because they can relate more easily to the erectile, visible part of the female than her invisible depths.

Sometimes a man is able to 'control' his ejaculation with his mind, by suppression, which a sensitive woman will experience as an interruption of the flow between them. Recovering the full flow and rhythm of the breath generates energy and authentic staying power. If the intercourse is rhythmical and relaxed the orgasm will rise from a depth that is beyond our wildest dreams, ending in genuine joy and possibly uncontrolled laughter, raising consciousness to a high level. Both partners feel freer and stronger, seeing life from a higher perspective, having experienced a true sexual communion culminating in the *glory of now*.

I think the essence of good sex is a capacity for genuine deep stillness and free energy flow, with a clear mind, an open trusting heart and harmonious breathing together, to allow for the *sexual energy dance* to happen.

I, personally, don't want to be less transformed by lovemaking than by standing on my head, otherwise I'll prefer to stand on my head for a half an hour, feeling connected and in one piece. I want lovemaking to enhance my connectedness not disturb it.

It is worth reminding ourselves that in lovemaking we may open to the earliest feelings of intimacy and the earliest hurt. Can I trust you with my heart? Can you trust me with your heart? It is a constant process of letting go of what stands in the way of being open and loving. If both partners are open to explore this journey then there is hope for true intimacy, for God's sake.

So what does it mean you can't have an orgasm?

Let's get down to the nitty-gritty:
It means fear.
It means holding on.
It means trying too hard while being tight deep inside.
It means not accepting your body fully,
It means you have internalised ideas about sex that made you close up.
Within the privacy of your own being learn to open your body.
Claim your freedom to let the energy flow through your body.
How?
Stop trying.
Become aware of the trying and do nothing,
Stop and relax.
Breathe deeply and rhythmically.
Learn the power of the full exhalation to surrender to the flow of the energy in your body.
Imagine all your cells smiling.
Feel how it lightens your internal weather.
Let your inner sun come out.
Be playful.
Laugh a lot!
Sing!
Dance!

*And we should consider every day lost
in which we have not danced at least once.
And we should call every truth false
which was not accompanied by at least one laugh.
Friedrich Nietzsche*

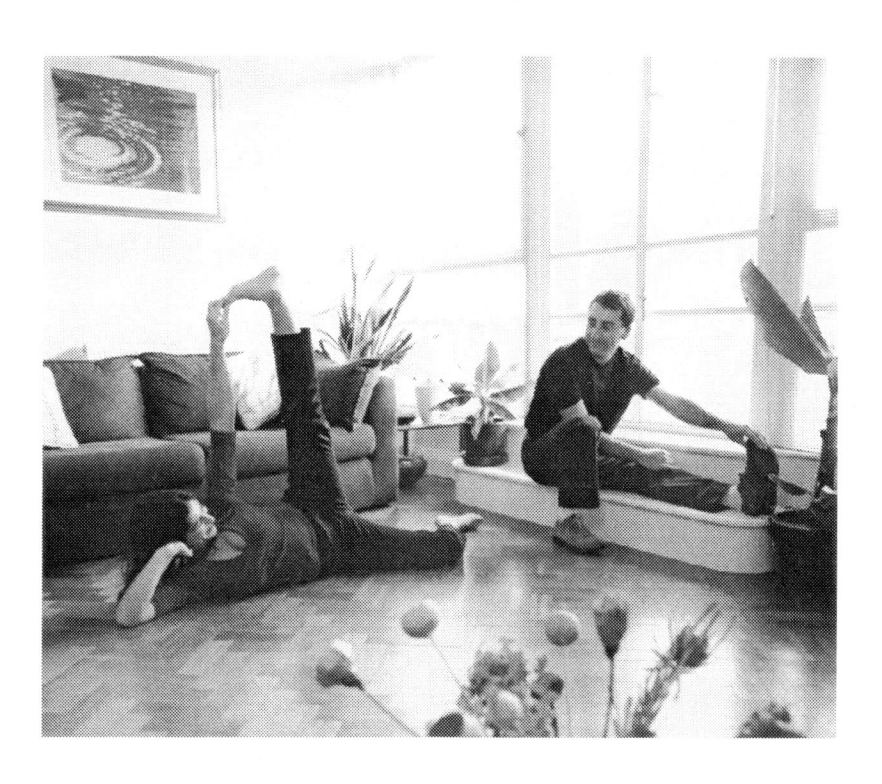

"What shall we do today, darling?"

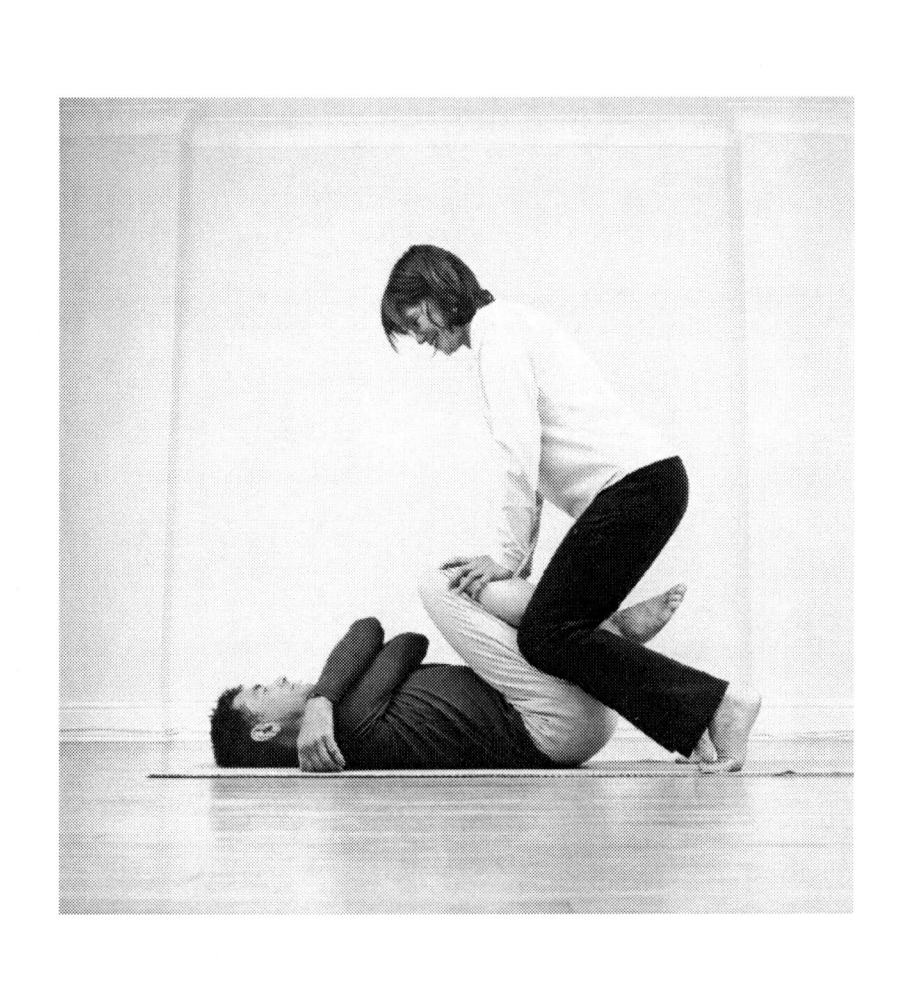

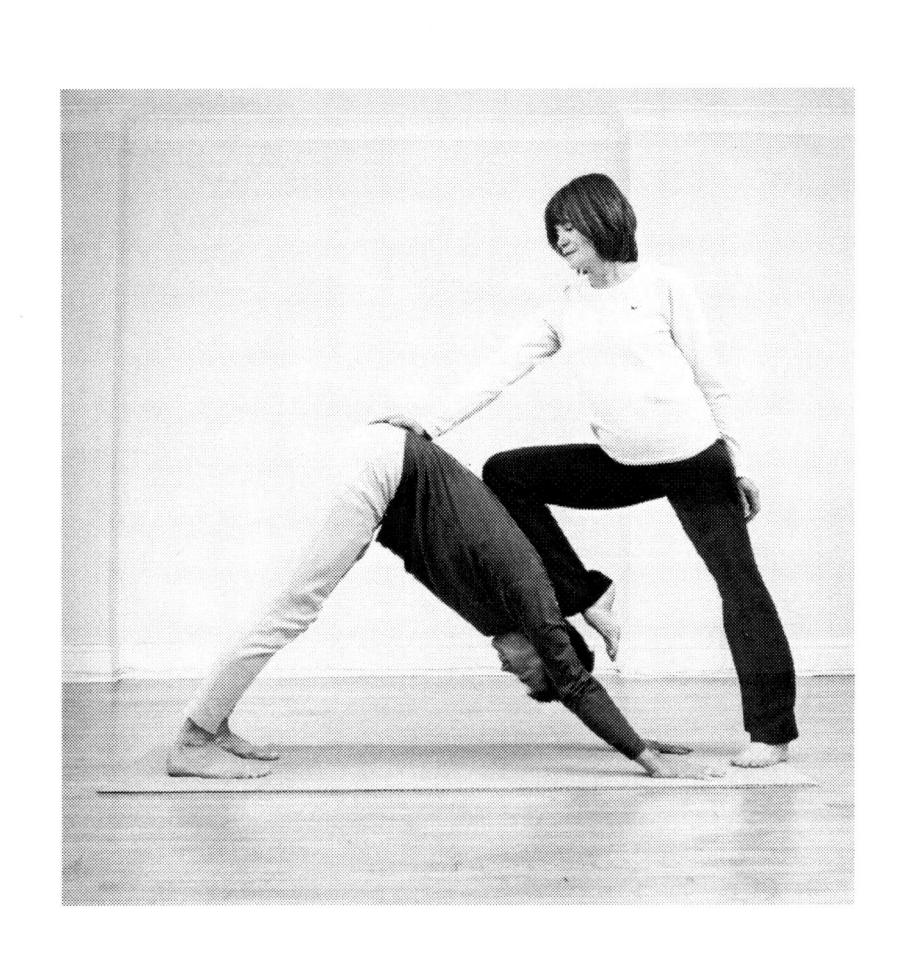

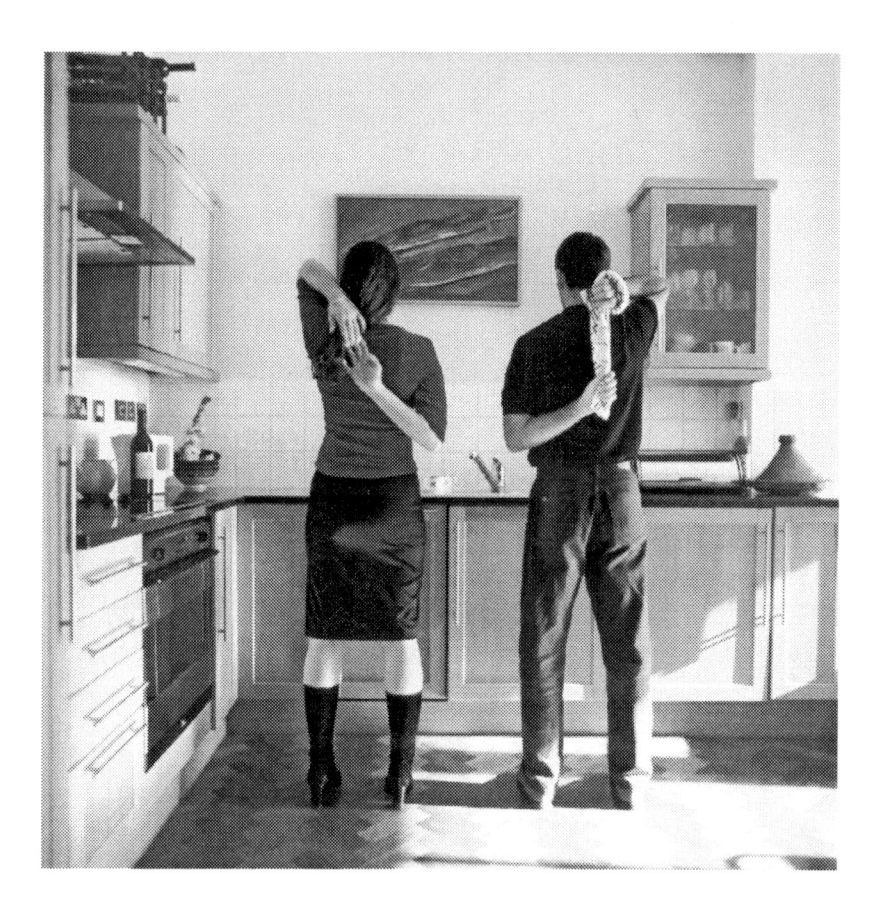

In the kitchen

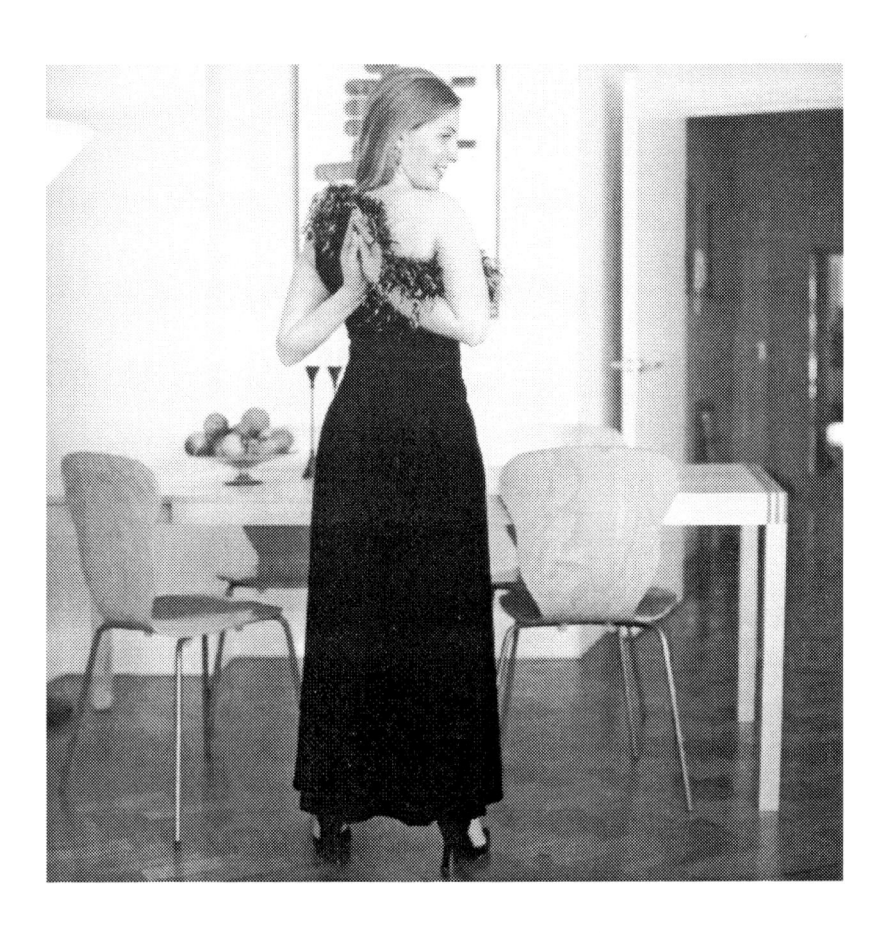

You don't have to disconnect at the party

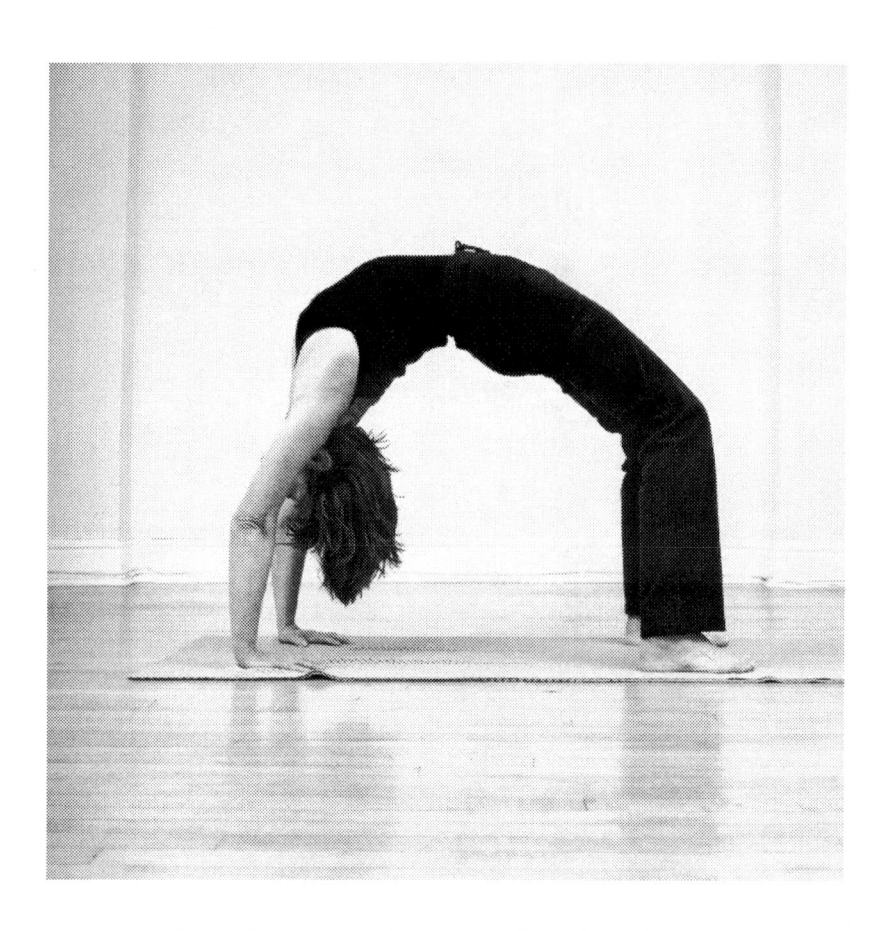

The older we get the more playful our joints!

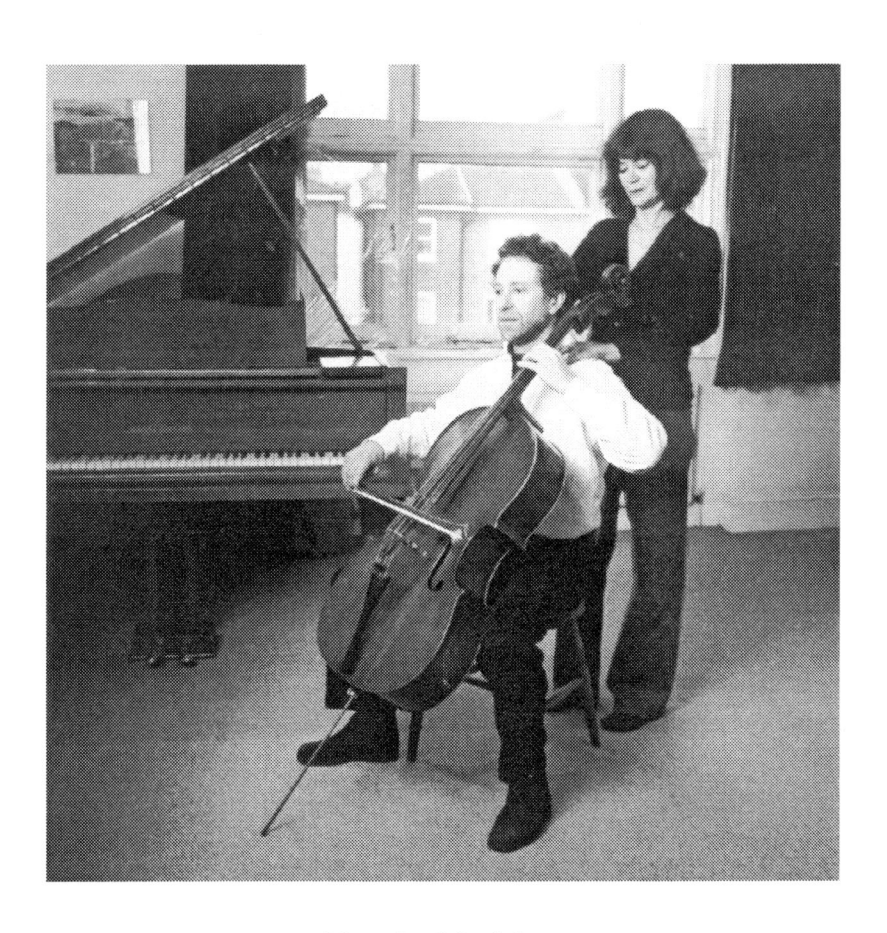

Yoga for Musicians

TWELVE

Teaching and helping others

'Here let me help you,' said the monkey, putting the fish up the tree.

To be of help to others we need to watch out not to put our hidden agendas onto other people in the name of helping. Ronnie Laing used to quote the Hippocratic Oath, 'Do no harm!', emphasising that one can do harm by 'trying' to 'do good'; he also said, 'One human cannot wake another up; the best we can do is not to sing lullabies to those who are waking up.'

My understanding of 'not trespassing' is having respect for the other's inner sanctum and sense of being. My aim in my classes is to create space for each of us to experience our presence together, giving us glimpses of faith, based on our own experience, that there is life beyond our habitual preoccupations. *Presence* is nearer to us than our breath.

Each individual unfolds and grows according to his or her own pace and rhythm, and the important thing in helping is not to get in the way of that unfolding. A good teacher will give instructions and encourage the confidence that is already within the student. I think that the only authentic help we can give is that of helping others to help themselves to get in touch with what's already there.

What do I teach and what lies behind the persona of a Yoga teacher?

I ask myself this question regularly so that I don't get stuck in any specific attitude. I don't want to have to pretend that I am beyond anger, fear, jealousy, envy, attachment to praise, fear of blame. It's too tiring to have to pretend. I practise relaxing with whatever I am feeling, letting go and at the same time, connecting to my centre, breathing and aligning my body in relation to gravity, as the good Lord intended.

If I honestly acknowledge and accept what is on my mind at the beginning of the class and don't try to change or manipulate it, relaxing and tuning in to my breathing rhythm, I notice that my heart opens and I am there for others in a genuine way. And that is what I like to share with others; becoming conscious of the body's alignment, of breathing, of how thoughts and emotions affect the flow of energy and how intimately inter-connected they are.

The first thing I am concerned with when I am working with others is to relax myself and not strain to help. How can I help another relax if I get all tensed up myself? Most of all I like doing nothing, in the spirit of Taoist *wu wei*, *effortless effort*, letting the creative energy flow through me whether I am working, reading, writing or helping someone else. I never make a plan but practise tuning myself up and if I am in tune the lesson flows. I notice how I tense up if I try to put a point across, if I am trying to change people.

I go through periods of asking myself, 'What am I doing teaching other people; is it a case of the blind leading the blind?' It is useful not to be afraid to ask this question. It deepens our connection to the source, taking us to the very root of our experience. I endeavour to stay at the source of creative energy and let it guide me; let it whisper in my ear.

Before each session I pray, 'If two or more are gathered together in the name of the truth, the way and the light, there the holy spirit shall be in their midst. May I be a channel for the healing of all the people present in this room and those who are absent'. And at the end of the session I say thanks and pray, 'May this session be of benefit to everyone present and absent and may I not take credit for the healing that sometimes happens.'

My classes are not about becoming stretch addicts. A good stretch is very pleasant and beneficial but the next minute you could be disconnected again! My classes are about awakening our awareness of the interconnectedness of our whole being. To be whole – healthy – to realise our 'being', requires nothing less than total surrender. This is the cream, the 'royal jelly' of the practice, if we dare to open our hearts and listen to our inner voice.

About teaching

'Thank you, master, for teaching me nothing.'
Taoist saying

'My education got interrupted by schooling.'
Bernard Shaw

The Masters say, 'Don't follow me, look within'. The Buddha said, 'Be ye lamps unto yourselves.' When I first read this it spoke to me in the most reassuring way. It implies a true respect for the autonomy and self-organisation of every being. The more we are in touch with our autonomy the deeper will be our empathy with each other.

One can feel lonely with other people. That loneliness of the soul that leads to the suffering of isolation has to do with being caught up in conditioned patterns, feeling a prisoner inside an isolated cocoon. Fear of accepting ourselves as we are keeps us isolated. We can only experience communion by being in the present moment where there is joy and love, and wishing each other well, something that can only be communicated through ease and kindness.

I invite all of us to come through our dark clouds to the clear space of letting the breath flow, feeling the ground under our feet, and opening our hearts.

THIRTEEN

Still more Yoga stories

Fidgeting

A man in my class says, 'This was a big achievement for me. I lay there for a few minutes without fidgeting.'

Stiffening up in the night

T. says, 'I feel more freedom in my hip joints. I feel more grounded in the root of my spine and my neck feels released. I am really happy about it…. aagh!.. but I'm going to stiffen up in the night and wake up stiff again.'

'It often happens that you experience relief from tension and then the tension springs back again. The force of old habits is very strong. That's why repeated practise is needed to get to the bottom of what's behind the habits and to make the relaxed state a more enduring and conscious.'

'But why should I get stiff during my sleep?'

'In sleep, when the cat's away the mice can play, the ego with its controlling power is asleep, so the emotional patterns from the unconscious emerge, affecting the body and the breathing patterns. If your emotional patterns are not resolved the body reacts by tensing up. That's why you wake up tense. In the morning it is essential to clear the effect of the night. Lie on the floor and relax. Wait for your breath to release and become more rhythmical, more harmonious.'

'Yes, they don't spend enough money on research about sleep. They don't understand sleep.'

'Whether *they* understand sleep or not, it's not necessarily going to help you understand why *you* wake up stiff after a night's sleep. The important thing is to keep getting in touch with your tensions and deeper emotional structures and release them consciously, then you'll be able to have a relaxed night's sleep and wake up refreshed.'

'Who's been driving my car?'

B. says, 'When I get into my car after a Yoga lesson I have to adjust the rear view mirror, because I sit straighter and taller. Sometimes I forget and wonder, Who's been driving my car?

Thank you.'

'My doctor says I am depressed.'

I think a state of emergency should be declared when people don't know what they feel and wait for the doctor to tell them!

Anxiety and depression are veils we put over our feelings. If we learn to get in touch with our feelings, recognise, acknowledge and stay with them we might be less likely to succumb to depression, or, if we are depressed, recognise that we are depressed and look at what lies behind the depression.

A. says, 'I am so relieved. The doctor said it's a virus. I couldn't understand why I've been feeling tired and run down for so long. It's such a relief!'

Yes, it is a virus, but it still doesn't absolve you of the need to be present to what was going on before you 'caught' the virus and after. Attending to and being honest about what is happening in your mind and body, and relaxing with it will prevent stagnant energy accumulating in the body where viruses have a chance to breed. Keeping the energy flowing strengthens your immune system.

First of all, let's be honest. It is self-deception that is responsible for most disease. How do *we* contribute to our unease? This is not blame! We have to touch our pain fully, make friends with it, accept it, without editing it, then it has it's own way of transformation. Books and wisdom don't help unless we apply what is being taught and make it our own experience.

'Is Yoga good for my immune system?'

'The peacock's splendour is his immune system'.
David Attenborough

Your immune system becomes weak because it is overburdened having to cope with stress. When your body is blocked all sorts of imbalances develop which stress your whole organism. Your organs literally get out of their orbit. If you can become attentive and present, feel your backbone and let your breath flow, all your organs will fall into place.

The basic principle for a healthy immune system is respect for the inherent balance of the body. You can't find it by thinking about it and manipulating it, you can only begin to touch on it by letting go of what is in the way of it.

It takes courage to be healthy because it means facing yourself honestly. In order to be truly healthy you must claim your inner ease. You need to think it through and realise that you don't need to be ill at ease if you take responsibility for your inner world. Yes, outer circumstances and other people affect your well being, but the ultimate responsibility is within you. Blaming other people for your irritations is not productive. Your immune system is intimately connected with how you respond to yourself, taking care to breathe and being connected to the ground, and not getting all stressed and out of it. The spirit in which you inhabit your body is your splendour.

Getting caught up in other people's energy while trying to help

L. feels that he carries the world on his shoulders.

'I can relax,' says he, 'but then there are so many people with problems, I feel sorry for them so I tense up again.'

'Tensing up is the easy way out. If you are frightened of your own feelings you dump them into your body and then think what a nice guy you are to suffer for your fellow men. To empathise with others does not mean taking on their problems and becoming as miserable as they are. If everybody did that there would be no one to turn to.'

He grins, 'You are absolutely right!'

'It's such a familiar scenario. In my childhood, everybody was always sacrificing themselves for others and then feeling tired and resentful and making others feel guilty at the sight of their uptight shoulders and sore backs. Only if we stop being frightened and endlessly running away from our own minds, can we listen to another and remain calm and a source of comfort and inspiration. Then the other person doesn't have to feel guilty that they have exhausted our resources. They can feel a restful place in us where they can refresh themselves like being in the shadow of a tree on a hot day.'

Grounding and breathing changes the quality of my life

A student phones, 'Mina, I enjoy your lessons so much, because of the space and time to experience the posture and the breathing. Grounding and breathing changes the quality of my life.'

Inner peace and stillness

One day in a class I say, 'During meditation we can touch inner peace and stillness.'

W. says, 'This is one thing I know nothing about. I only know how to spell it.'

Regret

'When I become more aware then I start feeling regret about all the things I did when I wasn't aware.'

'How could you climb a mountain if it were smooth? We need the rough edges in order to move on.'

The bud that wouldn't open

My Peace Lilly looked tough but it was only surviving, not thriving, in my basement flat. For years it never blossomed. One day, after all those years, I noticed a bud. I was overjoyed. It felt like a symbol for life finally unfolding and blossoming. Then weeks passed, a month passed, and still there was only a bud. I started to lose hope. But I did talk to it, sing to it, and gave it *Baby Bio*. One day it blossomed into this little umbrella-like white flower with a little yellow thing inside. It made me feel ashamed of my lack of faith.

D. says he hopes to be able to do a full lotus by the millennium. I told him the story of the bud. 'The opening happens from the centre not by physical manipulating.'

'And did it make you feel good?'

'Yes, I feel delighted, it's a thrill to see it. I thought it would shrivel up without ever opening. It confirmed my faith that flowering takes as long as it takes. You can't rush it. Or it's like pulling wheat by the stalks to make it grow faster.'

He asks, 'So how can my hips open?'

'Not by pushing your knees down, but by letting the tension unfold from the hips. Sometimes tension 'waits' till we get in touch with an emotional cause.'

'What kind of cause?'

'It could be circumcision?'

'Oh, yes.'

At the next session I say, 'We shall approach your groin from your head.'

'I like that,' he laughs.

'Meditate on the bud of the Peace Lilly. It takes time to create inner conditions of feeling safe enough to open. By not denying, not evading our feelings, the wholeness gets retrieved. It's like diving for pearls. The rational mind, if it's too dominant, tends to deny feelings. The reason for this is usually fear. By not denying feelings, learning to stay with your feelings, getting to know them you become less afraid of them. Only then can you relax deeply and the unfolding will happen by itself.'

FOURTEEN

Life is not a technique or a series of crises

> *'Man was made for joy and woe,*
> *and when this we rightly know*
> *through this world we safely go'*
> William Blake

*M*iddle age crisis, menopause crisis, old age crisis...
pre-natal crisis, post-natal crisis,
puberty crisis,
pre-menstrual crisis
post-coital melancholy

How is it that we make life into a crisis?

Growing in spirit, going through the stages of life with acceptance and dignity, enabling the latent spiritual power in us to manifest, moving from seeking power to authentic empowerment, living from the truth in our hearts is not easy or always comfortable.

To escape the discomfort we blame:
the weather
the full moon
the new moon
the half moon

a blue moon
PMT
SAD
TATT
POD

PMT – pre-menstrual tension.

Instinctively most women's bodies crave pregnancy, just like the soil 'craves' flowers to grow and blossom. But rational mind and circumstances don't always synchronise with instincts.

Before menstruation a woman might either be anxious that her period won't come, if she doesn't wish to fall pregnant, or anxious that it will come if she does wish to get pregnant. She might not be deeply conscious of those feelings. Lack of awareness of her feelings and thoughts, or running away from them, can create pre-menstrual tension.

There could be sadness with each menstruation that there has been no conception. If she is in touch with this sadness and melancholy maybe it doesn't have to turn into tension and anxiety, doesn't have to become a syndrome. It's just a normal cycle of the moon. Women in Egypt used to fast at each new moon and each full moon to stay in touch with the cycles of the moon.

In many traditions women spend time alone during menstruation in order to meditate, turn inward and surrender to the natural process of cleansing and renewal. If the circumstances of your life don't allow you to do this, make an appointment with yourself for ten minutes every day at least. Sit quietly, making a feeling connection with your body and your breathing and your particular story.

SAD – seasonally affected disorder

Sadness, which has been the sustenance of so much poetry, painting and music since time immemorial, the sadness, the poignancy of the changing seasons, has been turned into a disorder. How sad!

People get depressed when there is less light. Of course the quality of light affects us. But there is also truth in the fact that when we are unable to find our inner light we get more depressed by the lack of outer light. It doesn't seem to me that the outer light turns on the inner light; otherwise everyone in sunny countries would be enlightened!

TATT – tired all the time

I was alarmed to read in a newspaper about a condition called TATT, the latest phenomenon doctors are puzzling about. Is anyone considering the possibility that what makes us most tired is the toxic pollution deposited in our minds and bodies without the skill to cleanse it? If you get to know yourself and become honest with yourself, you'll learn how to cleanse your physical and mental energy channels, and you'll find that you are never tired.

TIT for TATT = NT - never tired, in touch with the creative flame of energy which is always there.

Cutting off from our feelings takes a lot of energy. If I feel agitated and pretend at all costs that I'm not, I will soon be exhausted. If I don't recognise my state of mind and how I am responsible for it, I will project my inner darkness onto other people or circumstances.

Whatever is happening in any situation can be an occasion to look at our reactions and behaviour. If I am able to acknowledge, 'I feel agitated and I'm breathing in, I feel agitated and I'm breathing out,' then I'm beginning to take responsibility for my state of mind, being present instead of cutting off.

By stifling our feelings, we stifle our whole being and become disturbed and tired and then say, 'It must be the weather.' You are feeling what you are feeling. Relax with it!

'Yes, but maybe I shouldn't be feeling it, maybe I'm wrong.'

'How can you be wrong to feel what you are feeling? Relax with your feelings and accept them. You'll create more tension by denying them. Breathe, so that you don't get into a knot.'

'But what do I do with all the feelings?'

'Observe them and accept them. They are your feelings, your barometer for what's going on for you. It is always empowering to relax with what you feel and not necessarily have to express it on the spot. If you deny what you're feeling, without reflection, your emotional reactions take control. A temper tantrum might bring temporary relief, but only until the tension accumulates again and you need another release, the way some people use sex.'

Waste of energy – Second wind.

What is *second wind?* Have you had the experience of feeling totally exhausted and then suddenly feeling a renewal of energy? What could be happening?

I believe that it means you've arrived at the total exhaustion of the muscles used to pull your centre of gravity upwards. Exhausted by the effort of the way you habitually hold yourself, physically and emotionally, you mercifully let up. So the *second wind* happens when you are so exhausted from pulling away from gravity that you cease to struggle and let your weary bones rest. Then the energy begins to flow freely through the channels.

Making mountains out of molehills or making molehills out of mountains

If our expectations and anticipations go ahead of our actions we are already using energy before we've even started. How often have I driven on the motorway, seen the traffic jam on the other side and worried all day about how long it would take me to get home only to find that by the time I was driving back it was the other way round! At least if I am conscious of my breathing, I can become aware of how my worrying is affecting it. If I have no experience of connecting to my breathing my physical condition will be continuously affected by something that hasn't even happened yet. My imagination has made a mountain out of a molehill and my body is flooded with unused energy.

We can use our imagination productively. For instance imagine your spine deeply rooted at the base and infinitely releasing upwards like a tree. Experiencing your body in relation to gravity will release the flow of energy. The more we can stay in the present moment, the more we can conserve our energy. The creative

rgy is always there whether we are tired or even ill, if
 and surrender to the source.

, Andrew Feldmar, a psychotherapist and writer, reminds that it's also possible to make molehills out of mountains, by underestimating the extent of hurt we carry inside. This can result in not giving, or not being able to give ourselves space to feel which, in turn can result in physical illness.

Self-fulfilling prophecy syndrome

When we perceive the present in terms of our past experience – when we have been disappointed or let down – our expectations and fantasies can lead to behaviour that could bring about precisely what we were afraid of. In that way our projections, of which we are not aware, can give us a distorted view of what's really going on, keeping us stuck in the same old habitual patterns.

To the degree that we are reluctant to look at our own responsibility, reluctant to make changes in ourselves to that degree we won't be open to allow the possibility of change in others.

Like this guy driving down the deserted country road in the middle of the night who suddenly gets a flat tire. He gets out of the car, looks in the boot and discovers that he doesn't have jack. What to do? He's cold, hungry and he must get home. Then he remembers passing a farmhouse a few miles back. OK, so there's nothing else to do but walk back there.

He walks and walks and while he walks, he starts imagining what might happen when he gets there. 'They might not be in …the farmer might not have a jack …he might be so angry at being woken up in the middle of the night that he might slam the door in my face. He might even have a gun…'

As he gets nearer the house he gets more and more worked up, more and more certain the farmer will be furious, refuse to help him and tell him to beat it. He continues to mutter to himself, 'The guy has no decency, no empathy, he's just a cold bastard…' and he knocks on the door, muttering away, and after a while the farmer comes out in his pyjamas.

And the guy shouts in his face, '…you mean son-of-a you can keep your fucking jack!'

'Opening up is scary.'

Physical blocks in the body often come about as a result of having to put up a defence against hurt, feeling unloved, unlovable, abandoned, rejected. The function of the armour is to block off feeling.

Before we can *heal* the trauma we have to *feel* it, become conscious of the defensive armour. Gradually, by breathing, practising full exhalation, we begin to unravel this defensive structure. To be able to exhale fully is to let go. If you can't exhale fully, the upper chest is all tight and pulled up. As you begin to let go your story that has been hidden in the armour for many years begins to reveal itself.

When you begin to let go of holding on, you begin to feel the texture of what you have been holding onto more and more. At that point it is tempting to go back into the same old defensive pattern, the armour might be uncomfortable but at least it's familiar. This is where it's so important to have support and encouragement to relax and stay calm with the emotional pain that arises as the tension gets unblocked and begins to dissolve.

A thirteen- year- old girl, B. who came for a Yoga lesson with her older sister, had the experience of doing a backbend and feeling a new opening in her chest. When she came out of it, she said, 'Oh, my chest really opened and it's scary'. She has scoliosis of the spine, her dorsal spine protrudes and her lumbar spine is extremely pushed forward, which is a way of sinking the chest in, trying to protect the heart. When I asked her, 'Do you tense up at school?' she said, 'No, everything is fine, I have no reason to tense up.'

At the next session she said, 'Yesterday I experienced relief and hope but now I am feeling worse again, not worse than when I first came but worse than I felt after the last Yoga lesson.'

I said, 'This does happen quite often. A release happens, then fear comes up, and the body tends to go back into its old familiar patterns. That's why it is important to practise regularly so that you can go through the resistance and fear and continue to open. Do you have trouble in saying how you feel?'

She said 'no' a bit too quickly and her sister looked at me and said, 'Of course she does.' At the end of the session she said, 'The pain in my back and shoulders is gone.'

She then chose an 'Angel card' - '*Openness*'.

She said, 'That's really cool. And it's scary.'

I asked, 'What is scaring you?'

She said, 'You just said to me that I should be able to talk about how I feel and that's what I feel, it's scary.'

She became conscious that she was afraid to say how she feels, and by admitting it she relaxed more.

The physical manifestations of our mental states...

...are expressed clearly in our body language if we open our eyes and dare to look at what we see:
> sunken chest - fear to open the heart;
> weak at the knees - inability to make decisions and follow them through;
> puffed up chest - centre of gravity pulled upwards, self-importance;
> weak spine - no backbone;
> chin in the air - leading with the chin- trying too hard, going against the grain;
> weak legs - no leg to stand on, no sense of a firm foundation in life;
> wobbly ankles - no support;
> elbow pain - no elbowroom.

What's wrong with sarcasm?

Sarcasm: *Ridicule; reproach; derisiveness; mockery; scoffing; disrespect.*

Oxford dictionary.

There are people who are habitually sarcastic without realising the harmful effect it can have. If your heart is open and you allow yourself to be vulnerable you'll feel the adverse effect of sarcasm in your heart. If we start paying attention to our heart and how it gets affected, then we might become more concerned with how we affect other people. Maybe this is where the first signs of stress begin.

The body in religion

I find myself wondering about how the body has been excommunicated from religion because of its desires and appetites. But surely until we can take responsibility for our own choices, there will always be an outside authority that has the final say? In some religions, a man is not supposed to look at a woman he is not married to, let alone touch her, not even shake hands. Surely if the body is busy keeping all desires under lock and key it's bound to be tense and uncomfortable. Is it not possible for a spiritual human being to act appropriately out of choice, moral, ethical, sensible choice, and not just rigidly obey rules?

Spiritual doesn't have to be dead – serious

Bob Monkhouse said, 'The only spiritual exercise I ever get is doing one press-up and saying, Oh, God.'

Our ability to laugh at ourselves is a powerful tool for cutting through our tendency to take ourselves too seriously. Clowns and jesters have always been part of tribal life in aboriginal societies. Instead of going to therapists people in conflict would go to a jester who, by reflecting back the troubled one's attitudes, would help them see the funny side of their pomposity and arrogance enabling them to let go, to resolve the conflict and connect again to the community.

To me being spiritual means becoming aware that I am part of a larger reality and that the universe doesn't revolve around me. It means joining my will with God's will, listening for guidance, for being moved to speak or do. It means being aware of my own impermanence and meditating on it, which helps me to feel compassion for suffering ...my own and others'.

True empathy is a spiritual quality. Periods of retreat and meditation in solitude are important in order to become more deeply grounded in the practice but it is the way we relate to other human beings and all of life every day that is the real arena. You'll be disappointed if you expect your third eye to open by closing the other two. 'Salvation' means 'safe return'. Return to your heart.

'Thy will be done' is the most difficult to practise. Somehow we feel that if we relinquish control, something terrible will happen. I suppose we'll no longer be able to deny death and that's what we're afraid of. It's easy to be a 'spiritual' person on holiday in a beautiful environment, feeling good and looking good with everything coming your way. But it's also possible that *when everything is coming your way you might be in the wrong lane!* It's when the disappointments come that it's much more difficult to accept them as part of God's will and to learn, from going deeply into the core of our discontent, to renew our purpose and say, 'Thy will be done.'

Love thy neighbour as thyself.

> *'Love is letting the other be, but with concern and affection.'*
> R.D. Laing

> *'All a sane man can ever care about is giving love.'*
> Hafiz

What really makes a difference to me is whether you listen to me with an open heart, acknowledging that fundamentally we are in the same boat; that we feel empathy for each other and that we can meet in our aloneness and companionship. Then we might find joy in our hearts. We are companions on the way, spiritual friends who are not trying to outsmart one another by our wit, intellect, and 'power clothes' or prove, 'I am right and you are wrong'.

The Distracted Centipede – a Yoga Exper.

If we can admit our vulnerability we can have a good laugh our predicament, how precarious our existence and what a joke that we are trying to hide it from ourselves and each other, rather than getting on with whatever it is we are doing, simply, from the heart. Our wits would become sharper and what a celebration there would be if all of us humans, can you imagine, would just drop hanging on to our puny identities, and have a song and dance.

This is what I understand by *'love thy neighbour as thyself'* …to wish other people what you wish for yourself …the gift of effortless being, in harmony with the laws of life, and with love in our hearts.

Ease comes from not having to pretend at all.

FIFTEEN

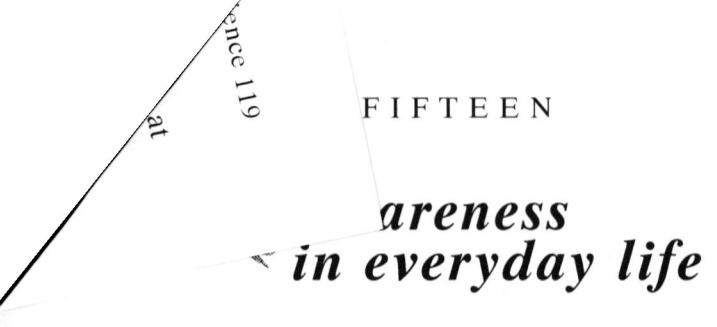

Awareness in everyday life

'Dear ones, let's anoint this earth with dance!'
Hafiz

'Take care.'

What are we talking about when we say 'Take care'?

> Take care not to fall under a passing car as you go out into the street.
> Take care to eat a good and balanced diet.
> Take care not to eat too much or too little.
> Take care not to sleep too much or too little.
> Take care that you are not too hot or too cold.
> Take care to take enough exercise.

But what about?

> Take care to let your breath move freely.
> Take care to let your shoulders drop away from your ears
> onto your shoulder girdle.
> Take care to let your spine be free and release upwards from its root.

Take care to feel the contact of your feet with the ground.
Take care to let your head balance.
Take care to have pleasure in movement letting your movements flow.
Take care to be more peaceful.
Take care to touch the inner stillness.
Take care to speak with kindness.
Take care not to be a danger to yourself.
Take care to be present.

There is always time

'I can never get going before that cup of coffee, not that I do get going, but I could get going if I wanted.'

Make an appointment with yourself first thing in the morning. Get out of bed and onto the floor to give yourself some time to unwind and centre yourself. Lie on the floor for a few minutes, letting your spine release and align.

Become quiet and aware of your breathing. Let it flow. You might become aware that your breathing is blocked and un-rhythmical. How do you let your breath flow?

Start from what you are aware of at this moment. Acknowledge what is on your mind; give yourself a lot of space with all your thoughts and feelings. If you are feeling sad, feel the sadness. You might feel sad but your heart and mind are connected.

You'll start feeling connected to yourself.

'I have no time,' many people complain.

There is always time. Be honest, you are looking for excuses.

When you are busy doing chores and the kids want your attention, and you feel distraught that you don't have the time to practise Yoga, think for a moment that you can bring mindfulness into whatever you are doing. You don't need any special time for it. How empowering is this thought!

Allowing just ten minutes in the morning to lie down on the floor consciously, to align your body, to take a few breaths, to make contact with gravity, to let there be space in your chest for your lungs and heart to function freely. To harmonise your breathing and to give your inner world some attention is at least as much a part of hygiene as spending hours deodorising yourself at the edges.

Even ten minutes of centering and breathing, lying on the back and letting the spine release, doing a simple spinal twist to release tensions accumulated in the night will do wonders for your health. It will make a world of difference helping you meet the uncertainties of the day ahead with courage, resourcefulness and good humour.

In the evening

Think back over the day, looking at the events and your own behaviour with as much honesty as you can muster, admitting mistakes and determining to correct them. Don't get stuck in regret; rather appreciate the lessons learnt from experience. We do inner work to become clear, but when clarity comes, it also reveals the things we don't like to see about ourselves. We have to remember that without seeing our shortcomings we can't begin to change them, so we eat some humble pie, acknowledge our transgressions and the pain they caused to others and ourselves, and hopefully don't repeat the same mistake. If we do make the same mistakes, which we do, we start all over again; acknowledge, accept, release, and let go.

That dissatisfied feeling.

Complain only that you are still complaining
Meister Eckhardt.

'The oyster shell fills not with pearls until it is content.'
Rumi

Here is the Queen of Jewish mother jokes: A waiter in a restaurant comes up to a table of five Jewish mothers out to lunch and asks, 'Is *anything* all right?'

Complaining and being dissatisfied about eve[rything is]
as much an addiction as drugs or alcohol. That dis[content]
lives obstinately inside no matter how many reassuran[ces you]
get that you are beautiful, attractive and loveable, or how many
material gifts you receive. It is an emotional response that might
have originated long ago and far away. Maybe from the moment
of conception or birth when you came out into the world and
people weren't sensitive to your needs when you were a helpless
baby, so that dissatisfaction set in and remained embedded deep
inside.

The way out of it is to get in touch with it by gradually peeling
off the layers of protective shell around you. Paradoxically, healing lies in feeling the wound fully.

Experience of contentment is one of the consequences of
Yoga practise. When certain conditions for balance are fulfilled
contentment arises spontaneously. Stay with what you are aware
of at this moment. However trivial or serious it may seem, let
your mind rest calmly on what you are feeling. Be compassionate
towards your feelings. It doesn't mean you approve of and agree
with your feelings, but that you allow space for them to come and
go.

Accepting the presence of what you dislike, staying with it
gently, breathing and contacting your centre can transform discontent into a mellow feeling of tenderness and gratefulness.

Being in the present moment is the best antidote to discontent.

The things you can always afford

> To smile
> To listen with heart
> Not to overeat
> Not to speak harshly
> To be kind
> To have a song in your heart
> To have a twinkle in your eye

Mina Semyon

In the kitchen

Become aware of how you stand in the kitchen while cooking or washing the dishes. You can save a lot of energy by simply being aware of your feet on the ground, dropping your shoulders and. breathing. Breathe while washing the dishes; breathe while cooking. Sometimes tenderness awakens and your heart opens just by taking care to wash a cup 'behind the ears'.

Waiting for the bus

Become aware of your feet and how they touch the ground. Don't worry; nobody can see you doing it. Let your weight go down into your feet, allowing your neck to relax. Let go of your head. Let your breath relax. At the same time acknowledge the surroundings. It won't make the bus come quicker but it will save you getting a headache and becoming irritable.

'Yes, yes,' you might say, 'It's all very well to be so smart if you don't have to stand in the freezing cold when you're late for work and the bus doesn't come.'

Life has a way of challenging our theories by presenting us with the opportunity to test them. I wrote the above before my car got stolen. After it was stolen I was given the opportunity to test my ability to relax while waiting for a bus on a drizzly Thursday morning and being late for a class.

I found myself thinking, 'OK, you've been talking about it, now show your mettle.'

And it wasn't easy. Some devil inside obstinately made me want to be restless and tense and irritable rather than do what I know is sensible.

So I said to myself, 'If you can't be sensible and reasonable and do what you know is best then be irritable, restless and tense. On the other hand if you can be sensible, relax, breathe and watch your emotions, then do that. The bus will come when it comes.'

Sometimes the best we can do is to be aware of how resistant we are to practising what we are preaching.

As a wise master said, 'The one who knows but doesn't act accordingly, knows imperfectly.'

Sitting in a car, stuck in traffic

Stuck in your car in endless traffic? Think, 'There is nothing at all I can do about it. If I give in to getting agitated, angry and frustrated I'll get more tired, get a headache, raise my blood pressure and most probably have an argument when I get home.'

For those who are capable of being reasonable for their own good, this is an intelligent thing to do. But how often do we know but go against what we know? When we will ever learn is hard to say, but hopefully when we observe the consequences of our own actions and look at them honestly, we'll learn from experience.

So …if you can …slow down, breathe out, make the exhalation longer. Feel your sitting bones in touch with the seat, release the spine between the shoulder blades, release your neck and exhale with a long hissing sound to help you exhale fully.

Make a sound, 'Ahhhhhh', like Marilyn Monroe in 'Ahhhhhh Wanna Be Loved by You'.

You might feel less inclined to hoot and shout at the person in front of you who is in the same situation, poor devil, and you might come home in a surprisingly good mood. It's not the situation itself that makes us irritable; it's our attitude to it.

Sitting in the dentist's chair.

Your head thrown back, your mouth wide open, the dentist's fingers in your mouth and the sound of the drill in your ears. Your neck is tensed, your shoulders hunched, and your breathing almost stops.

Not the most pleasant situation in the world, but why add more tension to it? See if you can possibly find it in yourself, even under these conditions, to try and claim your inner space. You might as well become aware of your contact with the seat, sink into it, become aware of your breath, which is tight in anticipation, and exhale quietly without being too demonstrative.

Acknowledge your fear. Say to yourself, '*This is fear*', and breathe out a long breath. Then breathe in from the lower abdomen and breathe out again.

It will relax the dentist, so he or she will do a better job, and you will avoid getting too much pressure in the head and neck, and remain centred as far as possible, under the circumstances.

At work

If people would only take the space to lie down on the floor consciously a couple of times a day for five minutes, to release the spine and let it find it's balance in relation to gravity, there would be less stress and lower back pain in the world! If there is no space to lie down then:

Stand next to your desk, put your hands on the desk with your feet apart the width of your hips and your heels slightly wider than your toes. Lean into your wrists, let your head hang; take a couple of long breaths. Then walk back till your spine is straight, feel your hips stretching away from your wrists, like two ends of a piece of elastic stretching away from each other. Keep your feet in line with the hips. Breathe out to the base of the spine, letting the shoulders relax.

Sitting at the computer

'I get very stressed working at the computer for hours.'
'Lie down on the floor for five minutes. Do the little twist.'
'I can't lie down in the office.'
'Then do the three way feet exercises. You don't need much space for that.'

In the shower

I asked a new student, 'How are you getting on?'
She said, 'I don't practise the postures yet, but I do pay attention to how I stand in the shower and I feel better straight away and also afterwards.'

After the gym

A student asked, 'What should I practice after a work-out in the gym?'

'Lie down on the floor with your knees to your chest, give yourself a hug, cross your feet the opposite way to your arms and breathe gently. Then cross your feet and arms the other way and again let go and breathe. This will allow your spine to release to its natural alignment, and release any tensions accumulated in the workout'.

At the airport

The plane is delayed, the departure lounge is chock-a-block with people and luggage, you are hot and restless, and your eyes are taking in too much movement and your ears too much noise.

The good news is that the outside commotion does not have to invade your whole being. Inner silence does not depend on the absence of noise.

Stop, just where you are, don't change anything, become aware of your feet touching the ground.

Become aware of your breathing.

Exhale deeply, feel your feet becoming more grounded, and your upper body releasing in response, like a tree.

Say to yourself, 'Calming my whole body I breathe in, calming my mind I breathe out.'

Jet lag

There is a story about a Red Indian chief who was being driven in a car at fast speed to a conference. After an hour he asked the driver to stop, got out, sat at the curb by the side of the road and just kept on sitting.

The driver asked, 'What's up?'

The Chief replied, 'I am waiting for my soul to catch up.'

Many people doubt that there is such a thing as a soul, but most people experience jet lag. Imagine the distances we cover while flying in a plane at tremendous speed of which we are not conscious except in theory. We've spent some time in a foreign place, met people and have a sense of that place in our body and mind.

By keeping conscious of all the stages of the journey and staying in touch with your breathing, you'll find the effects of jet lag will be milder, the coming down to earth smoother and the adjustment to the time difference easier. You'll find that you are together body and soul when you arrive.

Passing a driving test.

I learnt through experience that if I kept on studying and revising more and more in a nervous sort of state I'd be hopeless at passing my driving test. But if I created harmonious conditions in my body by staying mindful of my thoughts, practising letting them go and staying with my breathing rhythm, I'd become more balanced and relaxed. Then what I'd learned would be more accessible to me when I needed it. Before the test I practised Yoga, trusting that I'd learned enough and that it wouldn't run away if I relaxed. That's how I passed my driving test after failing it twice.

What does a handshake have to do with Yoga?

A handshake is a gesture of communication, a greeting. We shake hands in order to make contact, to exchange some good will. If we gain nothing from the gesture we might as well not do it. A handshake can communicate courage or weakness; fear of contact or a show of power that makes the other person's hand feel like it's going to fall off. Start by paying attention to the contact. You can't change that of which you are not conscious.

You don't have to disconnect at the party!

I think there is a popular misconception that being spiritual doesn't go with being glamorous and having fun. Glamorous doesn't have to be empty and superficial. Fun doesn't have to be flippant. You don't have to put on airs and disconnect from your centre because you are wearing fishnet stockings with red garters and a feather boa if that happens to be your whim at the moment.

The social pressure to be interesting

'Unheard melodies are sweeter'
Keats

The Distracted Centipede – a Yoga Experience

There is only one thing I find boring and that is the social pressure to be 'interesting'. There was a time when I used to have a notebook with jokes in it and before going to a party I'd memorise a few so that I'd have at least something to say.

It's fear of silence that makes your mind race, forcing you to think of something to say. And before you know it there is solid tension between you and the other person, emanating from your tense bodies. If we can just be together, giving each other and ourselves breathing space to be quiet and silent until we are moved by the spirit to say something - or not ...what a relief! Then there is a chance for something authentic to happen between us, even if it's '*only*' silence.

Try this exercise:

If in a social situation a thought comes up, 'I am not interesting, I have nothing to say,' say to yourself, 'I have nothing to say at this moment, I accept it, I breathe and relax. I just am, neither interesting nor uninteresting. I feel whole.'

If we could become comfortable with ourselves we wouldn't be afraid of silence and if we weren't afraid of silence we would feel comfortable.

If the musician was afraid of listening to silence the music would not have the uplifting quality of the spiritual dimension.

'Doing what comes naturally' doesn't need scientific validation.

It made my heart ache when I read an article by the scientific editor of the 'Independent' – '*Pigeons sniff the wind to find the way home*'. So they put the pigeons into an unnatural environment to prove that they lose their capacity to 'know the way home'.

Or, '*Bees can think, say scientists*' and do the same experiment on bees. What an insult to nature to have to trap these beautiful creatures, put them in unnatural conditions in order to prove that they lose their intelligence, which is otherwise intact when they are in their own environment.

Is it because we are out of touch with our inner magic that we don't observe with wonder and awe the intelligence of nature and celebrate it, rather than interfere with it?

Conscious eating

The spirit can't bear the body when overfed
and the body can't deal with the spirit
when underfed.
Aldous Huxley.

If you close your mouth to food
you can know a sweeter taste.
Rumi

My mother's greatest pleasures in life were to watch me eat or to fantasise about me marrying a millionaire. Since millionaires were even harder to come by than food in post-war Russia, as soon as rationing was over my mother really made me eat! So overeating became a device for cutting off painful feelings. When, for the first time in my life, I went on a fast of lemon and honey drinks for a week, I became free of the tyranny of my usual preoccupations and worries. I thought, 'This is it! This is enlightenment!' I felt calm and contented, filled with benign sensations in my body. After a few fasts I began to notice that in between feeling inspired and light, or dejected and lifeless, there was a loaf of bread with butter and jam!

I was inspired by these words from the I Ching :
Hexagram 27 - The Corners of the Mouth (Providing Nourishment)

Words are a movement going from within outward.
Eating and drinking are movements from without inward.
Both kinds of movement can be modified by tranquillity.
For tranquillity keeps the words that come out of the mouth
from exceeding proper measure and keeps the food that
goes into the mouth from exceeding proper measure.

Thus character is cultivated.

Proper measure? I found it easier to fast than to eat my proper measure. But eating as a means of relieving anxiety and insecurity destroys energy. There were times when the only pleasure in life seemed to be food, the only motivation to get up in the morning was looking forward to my favourite breakfast.

Graham Howe said, 'Suffering is digestion'. The stomach becomes overburdened and we become sleepy and lazy, there is an illusion of a relief from anxiety, in fact it is a dulling. The consequences are that we cannot achieve what we have set out to achieve. Gluttony leads away from communication to solitary gratification, which does not satisfy. I noticed there was a connection between believing in my dreams and losing that belief according to how much I ate. Then I came across a book *'The Huna code in religions'*, by Max Freedom Long, which confirmed my experience.

Max Freedom Long says, *'Kahunas believe that the seat of the low self was in the intestinal tract and the low self is the place where fixations and convictions of unworthiness and guilt must be sought and removed.'*

Maybe that was one of the reasons why my mother kept urging 'eat, eat, my child'. Guilt had to be fed and kept alive at all costs!

It is a deep-seated problem, this overeating, and a very common one, and yet there isn't a quick solution. To change this monster habit on a deep level is to discover it's root, by doing the inner work and to realise how deeply our relationship with food affects the balance of the body and mind. Getting in touch with the sense of balance and becoming more attuned to it makes us more reluctant to lose it through overeating or eating unconsciously.

How can we change our eating habits?

Practising Yoga with mindfulness helps to awaken and to trust our intuition so that we know when to eat, what to eat and how much to eat. If we are in touch with ourselves we don't need to be told by experts what to eat.

Yogis advise not to eat until the breath flows freely through the right and the left nostril. In the physical and subtle bodies there are a certain number of *nadis* (subtle channels through which energy flows) and *chakras* (centres in which cosmic energy exists).

The nadis emphasised in Yoga are *ida, pingala* and *susumna*. In most people the nadis are obstructed but asanas and pranayama can clear them. *Ida* and *Pingala* represent the sun and the moon, the right is the sun, the left the moon, the male and female principles. *Susumna* is the central channel in the spinal column and is regarded in Yoga as the road to *nirvana*, which means cessation of all the spinning in the mind. To breathe freely through the right and left nostrils is to unify the two breaths, and free the central channel.

Alternate nostril breathing is a simple and important exercise for our digestion and general health to practise every morning before eating.

Getting rid of headaches without drugs.

Lie on your back on the floor, legs over a couch, buttocks touching the edge, arms by the side relaxed. Put a book under your head and with your hands lengthen your neck. Close your eyes, put two small rice pads on your eyes, let your eyes relax into your eye sockets, imagine your eyes like two pebbles sinking into a lake till they reach the bottom and become still. Breathe gently, become aware of and let go of thoughts. Feel the lower back sinking into the floor. Imagine the tension in your neck and shoulders, hip joints and legs melting away. Lie like this for ten minutes and enjoy the difference.

Forgiveness

'Oh I am not there yet, maybe when the sun begins to shine, and the weather gets warmer,' said J. when I mentioned forgiveness.

Forgiveness rises out of your heart as a consequence of having gone to the rock bottom of the pain of alienation that non-forgiveness creates, not because you are in a good mood. It's easy to forgive when you are feeling good, but the resentment will come back when the clouds obscure the sun again.

Forgiveness is realising that we are all in the same boat. It is wishing for oneself, as well as for everyone else, that we may be able to redeem our past mistakes and ignorance.

Making mistakes is part of our learning. Not being able to forgive yourself is a device to stay in the same old clutches. Being able to forgive yourself means facing the truth about yourself and moving on. We need to forgive ourselves and even those who don't forgive us.

Robustness

'If you take umbrage at every rub how will you become a polished mirror?'
Rumi

In Yiddish umbrage, a sense of slight or injury, is called *'farible'*. In my childhood everyone was always keeping a 'farible'. No wonder everyone was always complaining of ailments, 'akh, akh my back, oy, oy, my knees'. How can your body relax if it's full of faribles?

I believe that our task on this earth is to become loving, open and joyful human beings capable of celebrating life. For that we need to clear our physical and emotional channels of accumulated dross, outmoded beliefs and cliché expectations.

'But we know that the leopard doesn't change its spots.' This statement is an illustration of the clichés we carry inside us, without realising how trapped we are by them. People don't change because it takes courage and humility to accept ourselves as we are, which is the starting point.

*When we acknowledge and accept our conditioned
emotional patterns,
even accept the resistance to accept them,
we come into the spaciousness of the present moment.
We become tougher and not so precious and touchy about our
fragile egos that can't take a drop of truth without falling
apart or becoming aggressively defensive.*

'The hardest person to wake up is the one who thinks he's
already awake.'
Mahatma Ghandi

SIXTEEN

Yoga and the Ageing Process
The older we get the more playful our joints!

'I'm not ageing – I'm ripening to perfection'
Anonymous

The good news is that our joints don't have to become rigid through ageing. Scientists have discovered that DNA has a capacity for self- repair and that it is also influenced by our every thought, feeling and action.

Yes! By paying attention to your mind, body and breath, and their interrelatedness, you can become lighter, freer and healthier, and your immune system, stronger. By tuning in to your inherent balance you can create ease and conditions for healing. Your joints can become playful with age!

Imagine! You step out of your own way and let your body do it's magic! It will work effortlessly and harmoniously. If we could just drop all the resistance we'd feel free, but since we often can't, we have to keep getting in touch with the resistance and letting go of it gradually by degrees.

And if you can let go in one leap of faith, good for you!

Getting the grannies out of the groin

See if you can begin to enjoy being in the moment, being mindful, whether you're sitting, standing, lying down or walking.

Then you might get the potential for hot flushes out of your groin even before the menopause. That's where they have been hiding in women for generations, in socially imposed limitations and inhibitions.

Get your grannies out of your groin. It's never too late and never too early. We are all flowers in different stages of unfolding.

Menopause is not a disease unless you make it into one by resisting the natural process. Let the energy flow, menopause or no menopause. Menopause doesn't have to be meno-poisonous.

Free your groin, inhabited by the ghosts of many generations not allowed to feel their bodies, not allowed to swing their hips. Get your grannies out of all your nooks and crannies! Evict them! Let them join in the great cosmic dance. That's what we can do for our ancestors- release them.

When I say this in a class most people laugh spontaneously, but occasionally someone asks, 'what kind of Yoga is that?' What I mean by 'grannies in your groin' is all the conditioning that got lodged in there over generations, the groin being a particular place for storing sexual inhibition.

Each generation has the responsibility to liberate itself a little more from traditional fixed ideas. Tradition!

'But what about honouring my ancestors?'

'Maybe the best thing we can do to honour our ancestors is to let them out of our body and set them free.'

We would need a lot less medical interference and the National Health Service wouldn't be so overloaded if we could just become aware and let go of some of the inhibiting conditioning that is blocking our energy flow.

'How does becoming aware help?'

If you knew you were digging your nails into your palm wouldn't you be foolish to keep digging them deeper? If you are not aware of doing it you will go on even though it's obviously self-destructive. So who can argue with that?

And don't worry about what kind of Yoga this is. Call it 'Sensible Yoga', or 'Basmati Yoga'. Often what it is called becomes more important than the experience of it. First experience it and then see what you want to call it. This is what those Yogis did. They just practised and practised in the forests in India and then expressed what they experienced and passed it on to us, which is great. All the same we have to find our own experience of Yoga, otherwise we are hooked into dogma. It becomes a case of 'My *karma* has just run over your *dogma?*' Have a laugh. Your sense of humour is intimately connected with freedom in your body. Laugh from your belly!

Menopause.

'Ten thousand flowers in spring
the moon in autumn
a cool breeze in summer
snow in winter
If your mind isn't clouded
by unnecessary things
this is the season
of your life'.
Wu-Men 1183-1260

Does this year's spring regret being so much older then the spring of many years ago? 'Oy, I was so much younger then.'

In autumn, does the birch tree knit its brow and get anxious when autumn leaves start to fall?

Growing old? The important word, surely, is *growing* and we never stop growing. Maybe we don't have to turn life into a series of crises if we stay present and go with the flow through all the different stages of life.

Women are forced into the collective image of what it means to be a post-menopausal woman. A woman of any age can be a going concern in all her compartments if she stays in tune with the life in her, as well as all the anxieties and despairs. As Mae West said, 'It's not the men in my life, it's the life in my men.' If you let your energy flow your honeyed secretions don't have to dry up because you are no longer nineteen.

All the herbs and diets in the world won't help if we don't know how to slow down and 'go with the flow'. Ignorance is going against the flow and not even knowing that there is a flow. We dig our heels in, resist life as it is and wonder why we are feeling out of it. And then *blame it on the Bossa Nova!*

If we become conscious of our feet on the ground and our spine releasing from the root upwards, let our head balance and allow our breath to flow, we'll experience wholeness and youthfulness, at least for a moment. Let such moments accumulate!

And sometimes I personally 'lose it'. Who doesn't? But I don't feel that because I still lose the plot from time to time it devalues my insights or makes me into a fraud. If habitual patterns still come up I hope to be able to recognise them. The practice I am talking about helps to develop skills to notice and to deal with what comes up, helps to make us less frightened to let it come up, to 'lose it'. If we are not frightened of 'losing it' we don't have to hold onto it and we might eventually realise that there was nothing to hold onto and no need to hold on in the first place!

The other day I was shopping at 'Fresh and Wild' organic food shop. As I was paying, the assistant said, 'Do you know that as a mature citizen you are entitled to 5% discount?'

To be honest I would much rather have paid the full price than be recognized as a mature citizen!

'I am tired,' I caught myself thinking, 'I don't look my best.'

Akh! All this trying to hang on to the illusion of being young and still attractive to the opposite sex for one more day, and missing out on being who I am at this moment and the wisdom that comes with it.

It's much more practical to cultivate awareness of life beyond our disturbed and disturbing minds, opening the way to a more balanced, rhythmical, supple way of being, no matter what age.

When someone says to you, 'You look so young today', is it really a compliment? So, at other times I look old?

When a young actress said to Mae West at her seventieth birthday party, 'Darling you don't look seventy', Mae West replied, 'This is what seventy looks like!'

It's really weird, the stigma attached to being a woman of a 'certain age'. It is a very uncomfortable feeling. Suddenly you feel you are being labelled, isolated, put into a category, put in a box. It's quite a scary feeling, not unlike racism. You are being treated in a certain way, which has nothing to do with who you are. So yes, it helps to practise mindfulness and Yoga with breathing, so you don't get caught up in the image others project on you out of their own needs and limitations. To me Yoga has been a way of becoming more confident in the inherent common sense of my being so that I can stand up against everything that demeans the dignity of life.

How can death be bad for you?

'I am not afraid of death, I just don't want to be there when it happens.'
Woody Allen.

Paradise –
I see flowers
from the cottage where I lie.
Yaitsu's death poem, 1807

In my childhood in a suburb of Moscow death was a nasty subject, to be hidden, not to be spoken about, to be avoided at all costs, creating tension, unease, disease, so we were already more dead than alive.

When my mother heard someone had died she used to spit three times over her shoulder, *'tsfu, tsfu. tsfu'* and say, '*It shouldn't happen to us*'.

Occasionally when a Communist Party member died they carried him in an open coffin through the streets, accompanied by brass wind instruments playing window- rattling funeral marches.

My mother would rush to close the windows trying to protect me from the extreme grief that every reminder of death had provoked since my father died when I was four.

We human beings think we are different from everything else on earth. But everything is born and dies and we sort of know it applies to us as well, but 'we have such a superior intelligence we must find a way out of this predicament'. We just can't come to terms with it and live and let live while we are still alive. When I first heard about the Buddhist contemplation on death I couldn't even imagine getting started.

Learning how to let go continuously can allow us to go through the stages of life as a natural process, including ageing and dying. Dying could then perhaps be akin to a leaf falling from a tree. Yes, it is sad to realise the impermanence of everything and everybody near and dear including ourselves. So we can begin by relaxing with the sadness, which will open and mellow our hearts.

'Oy, am I stiff,' people say, but who says,
'Oy, my heart is closed, I can't feel sadness, tenderness, love, sorrow.'

> If you can relax with your feelings,
> You can be sad and relaxed.
> You can be sad and not depressed.
> You can feel fear and not be afraid of feeling it.

There is a private joke between airline staff when they talk about safety on board and suggest that in case of emergency you put your head between your knees. 'Put your head between your knees,' they say over the loudspeaker, and then, to each other '...and kiss your arse goodbye!' So maybe this is one of the advantages of becoming supple through the practice of Yoga.

> *'I died as a mineral and became a vegetable.*
> *I passed away as vegetation and became animal.*
> *Leaving the animal state I became Man.*
> *Why should I fear?*
> *When was I less through death?*
> *I shall once more die from manhood to soar with angels,*
> *and I must go beyond angelhood - all perish but God.*
> *When I have given up my angel-self, I shall be what no mind has conceived'.*
> **Rumi**

SEVENTEEN
...and still more Yoga Stories

'Before we start the Yoga...'

S. talks about her relationship to her illness, 'I'm having orthodox medical intervention but I am also addressing it from a holistic point of view. Through my illness I am becoming more aware of how the illness has come to be, that it is a consequence of accumulated denial of pain and hurt in childhood which I've never addressed it in an embodied way.'

'I am having acupuncture treatments and homeopathy. I find it hard sometimes to withstand the conventional doctors diagnosis and prognosis. I need to find courage, without being reckless, to stand my ground. I am actually getting better and feel that in the long run it will be Yoga and increasing awareness that will heal me.'

While she talks I sit on the floor cross-legged, keeping up awareness of my contact with the ground and breathing which doesn't diminish the quality of my listening and being present, on the contrary it makes it sharper. She is also sitting on the floor but I can see from the way she is sitting that she is not applying what she knows to the sitting posture while she is talking. Somehow the sitting and the talking seem separate.

Then she says, 'One more thing,' in a tone that implies, 'before we start the Yoga.

I say, 'There is no separation between 'the Yoga' and what we are talking about now. While you are talking you can still be aware of your breathing and contact with the ground. You said earlier that you've been feeling good but it doesn't last. Suddenly for no good reason you are feeling bad again. I believe that connecting your awareness with ordinary activities, by letting this connection grow and become stronger your sense of well being will become more consistent.'

Husband and wife

Teaching Yoga to a mother and a daughter in the master bedroom of a suburban mansion.

The husband comes in, watches the class for a few minutes and says to his wife, 'I'm glad that for a change you have to do what someone else is telling you to do.'

Go organic.

'I can't 'go organic', my husband goes potty when I mention the word organic.'

'You don't have *to go organic*. Just buy, cook and eat organic food.'

'Haven't thought of that'.

I love Yoga

N. says with great enthusiasm, 'I love Yoga. Just to be able to sit on my heels is a big achievement. I now dry my hair sitting on my heels. I can now bend down and squat to get something out of the bottom of the refrigerator. Or if my daughter spills something I can now bend down without any trouble and wipe it up without getting irritable with her.'

Yoga — a way of dissolving defences.

After a Yoga class J. looks at me with tears in her big blue eyes and says, 'I didn't realise that in Yoga practice defences begin to dissolve and old pain gets revealed.'

'...and all this you learnt from Yoga?'

T. sits on the floor with his legs stretched out in front in the Yoga posture *Parshchimotanasana*.

I say, 'Follow your breath and allow the muscles in your legs to relax, so that they can release to the floor. Feel how the tension in your legs is pulling them up to the ceiling. Breathe and let gravity relax them down.'

T. tries to push his legs down with his hands, tightening his shoulders in the process.

'I need two sandbags to hold my legs down.' he says.

'Sandbags are a temporary solution. Breathing and releasing consciously is the more lasting one. It will get you in touch with what makes you hold on. Feel your legs making contact with the ground, let the contact get deeper.'

'No, I need two sandbags.'

I go and lie across his legs like a big sandbag, breathing and enjoying myself.

He relaxes for a moment.

After a while I get up.

T says to his friend, 'It's great to have a woman lie on top of your legs like this and not feel any pressure to have to do anything.'

'Yes, in intimate situations the pressure to do something is often an obstacle to allowing the spontaneous closeness to happen. If only lovers could breathe deeply and freely they would move naturally to sexual intimacy. It would open before us a thousand and one nights of wonders and delights beyond our wildest dreams. Fidelity would become a natural condition, if both partners would engage in the process of seeing each other and themselves with fresh eyes, which is the meaning of respect.

Sex life would have that quality of the unexpected and new without trying to contrive it with sexy underwear, not that I am against sexy underwear. Eros resides in tenderness. We don't need pornographic magazines or videos to turn us on, if we relax and let it happen. One relationship could remain an adventure for a lifetime ...I think.'

'And all this you learnt from Yoga?'
'Yes'.

Accepting is not the same as complying

'Lie on your back, with knees bent, your feet on the floor about a foot apart. Become aware of your body being aligned; neck in line with the spine, hips in line with your shoulders, feet in line with your hips. Give yourself a big hug, open between the shoulder blades, leave your arms crossed and relax your wrists, let your hands hang. Do nothing.

Start by acknowledging where are you at this moment? Acknowledge your thoughts and emotions, however trivial they seem, don't censor anything, let it be, give yourself space, accept yourself with all the thoughts and emotions and physical sensations. If you don't accept where you are at this moment how can you move on? Accepting is not the same as complying.'

'How is it different?'

'*Accepting* means acknowledging not denying. Acknowledging is a starting point; it's an entry into your being. Register, reflect and release. *Complying* means to act in accordance with, give in and give up, fit in, know one's place.'

'I see the difference.'

She had to give up a high-powered job because of chronic tiredness. She was at first highly sceptical that her thoughts might affect her body or that her physical condition was actually connected with her tendency to 'get frenetic' as she put it.

'Don't you think being frenetic is what is making you tired?'

'But how?' she demanded.

'Getting frenetic is like making mountains out of molehills, your body is using energy far beyond the task at hand. If you can learn how to slow down and connect to your body and your breathing, you'd save a lot of the energy you are using unnecessarily.'

After six months of lessons she was able to go back to work but found that she still got tired and had to lie down at lunch time in the rest room.

'I fall asleep immediately, and feel rested, but after a while I feel tired again.'

'If you continue learning how to relax inside yourself more you won't be using unnecessary energy. That's what makes you tired.'

'But how? I feel very passionate about my work.'

'You don't need to give up your passion and commitment; you just need to become calmer inside. You can become more relaxed about what you believe in, you can express your views with passion but without getting wound up and tight. Maybe because you weren't properly 'heard' in childhood you've developed a habitual way of talking to 'deaf ears'. It's like talking to the wall, you might be anticipating not being heard so you have to push too hard'.

'Yes, that rings a bell.'

'Listen to your voice while talking, feel the ground as you are listening, feel your breathing, maybe hear a bird singing at the same time. Listening doesn't have to be stressed and narrow, it can be relaxed and open.'

'Yes, I get very frenetic and probably make other people nervous.'

'If you could relax and speak from a calmer place then you would give the others space to relax and make it easier for them to hear you.'

'But how do I do that?'

'Become quiet and recognise what is making you uneasy at this moment. Recognise it and accept it. Relax with yourself as you are and you'll feel your breathing relaxing into a flow and you'll feel a deep sense of release.'

'Can you say again how accepting is different from complying?'

'Acceptance means acknowledging that you are feeling uneasy and that you are straining to push your point across; that you are getting frenetic and you are not aware of your breathing and haven't been aware of contact with the ground for a long time. It requires courage and honesty. Accepting that this is what is happening means you can do something about it.

Compliance means, *That's how I am. It's genetic; it runs in the family. My mother was like that and therefore there is a good reason why I should be the same, it's Pluto, it's Venus, it's my Saturn return, there's nothing I can do about it - so I'd better go along with the collective consensus or I'll be left out.* That's complying.

By accepting, letting go and staying open we meet in communion not in collusion.'

'Yes, I can see the difference.'

'Wouldn't it be lovely if it were possible to introduce breathing awareness into work places for all the people who don't know how to relax?'

A relaxed dentist

A dentist in my class said, 'It's all very well talking about being at ease and letting go, but I can't do it when I am leaning over patients all day long.'

'Wouldn't it be wonderful to have a relaxed dentist?'

Someone else said, 'I once had a relaxed dentist and he was useless.'

Of course you don't want a surgeon who is cool and laid back at the expense of his skills. It's a fine balance between being relaxed and acutely present at the same time.

In the beginning most people fall asleep during relaxation after a Yoga class because it's very hard to maintain this fine level of being relaxed and alert at the same time. Most people associate alertness with being stressed.

High- powered means that you are expected to be wired. In fact you are most alive and vital when you can let go and relax allowing all the functions in the body to do their job effortlessly. When we get out of the way then vitality is there at it's highest.

It is actually possible to do Yoga for years and years and years and still not be able to extend what we've learnt into our everyday life. Yoga can also become part of our ego baggage that we carry around on our shoulders.

So to really clear out the old baggage takes time and patience, honesty, courage and perseverance to keep going. From my own experience of doing Yoga for thirty odd years I find that the same old emotions and states of mind keep recurring but being able to get in touch with the inner centre enables me to acknowledge them quicker and let go quicker - and sometimes not.

EIGHTEEN

Take as long as it takes

> *One can never become a Buddha*
> *One can only discard the illusion*
> *that one was ever anything else*
> A Zen saying

How long will it take to remember to remember?

R. sits on the floor with her legs stretched in front to bend forward and touch her feet. She strains, she loses contact with the ground, pulls up into her shoulders and neck and alarmingly holds her breath. I suggest she take a breath to relax her shoulders, get in touch with the ground and let the base of the spine become grounded.

'Exhale to the bottom of the spine and, from above the waist, let the whole body release, so that reaching to the feet is like a plant growing towards the sun with the roots growing deeper into the ground.'

After the class she thanks me, 'I've really learned something important. The problem is how to remember?'

'Remember to take a pause, to get in touch with your breath and gravity when you are doing a posture. If you start straining and using will power, remember the breath and let it guide you into the posture'.

I remember, years ago, when I first started to become aware of my mind and body and discouragement was lurking around every corner, how I used to write at the end of my shopping list:

Milk
Butter
Vegetables
Fruit
Flowers
Don't forget to thank God

I thought that if I practised thankfulness, even if I didn't feel it, it might become real in the end. If you can't make it, fake it.

Eventually thankfulness started to replace discontent more often when I managed to remember that there is no end to discontent. If it weren't for forgetfulness we'd always remember. Remember that you forget to remember. Recognise it as soon as possible. When you sit down and become quiet remembrance comes.

Conversation with Rifke in her garden

'How are you?'
'My heart is heavy.'
'My heart is heavy and I breathe in. My heart is heavy and I breathe out.'
'Oh but it's so dense and tense.'
'It's dense and tense and I breathe in, it's dense and tense and I breathe out.'
'I am feeling insecure.'
'I am feeling insecure and I breathe in I am feeling insecure and I breathe out.'
Pause...
'It feels lighter.'
'It feels lighter and I breathe in.'
'It feels lighter and I breathe out.'
'But how can I remember?'
'Remember to remember.'
'What am I trying to remember?'
'Not to forget.'

A student in my class asked, 'How long will it take for me to become supple?'

I replied, quoting Patanjali's Yoga sutras:

'Success varies according to whether the effort is mild, moderate or intense.
'Success is immediate where effort is intense'
and *that* was said sometime between 200 BC and 200 AD.'

How long will it take before we stop looking for love everywhere other than in our own hearts?

Like Mula Nasrudin looking for his keys under a lamp post. Someone asked, 'Is this where you lost them?'
'No', replied Nasrudin, 'but it's lighter here.'

Imagine! There is a magnolia tree, symbol of inner and outer peace, *the* flower of patience, which blossoms only every sixteen years.

How long will it take to stop waiting for everything to be all right before we start breathing freely?

How long will it take to stop denying the muddy patches we need to go through?

Like the cartoon of God parting the Red Sea to let Moses and his people pass from Egypt to the land of milk and honey, from darkness into light, from bondage to freedom.

All the people are standing hesitantly on the shore and Moses is saying, 'What do you mean, it's a bit muddy?'

Practice of Yoga changes our relationship to pain — it becomes something to go through rather than to avoid.

I've noticed that being able to stand on my head for half an hour, or do a 'sensational' back-bend, making some people gasp with admiration, (which is what I was doing it for!), didn't increase the love in my heart. In fact, in the beginning it increased arrogance and pride.

So what did start awakening love in my heart?

Oh, living and suffering and gradually realising that being constantly preoccupied with myself leads to isolation and loneliness.

Becoming aware of self- deception and developing a taste for being honest with myself.

'The Cloud of Unknowing' advises us to *'think of a Cloud of Forgetting between you and your sin* (*sin* in this sense of *missing the mark*)*, and a Cloud of Unknowing between you and God'*. It feels reassuring that God and love cannot be defined or known by thinking.

You can only know what love is not. It is not judging, it is not holding grudges, it is not being competitive. It is not in one-upmanship, it is not in boasting. It is not in putting on airs; it is not in trying to impress. It is not in being arrogant; it is not in being divided.

Sometimes we want to give up in despair because it seems impossible to let go. And then something shifts and lets in a chink of light and it all seems all right again. Or, as Christopher Robin said about Winnie-the-Pooh, 'Silly old bear.' And everyone felt hopeful again.

This is what I've been doing for the past thirty odd years. Working on the mind-body in a way that deepens the awareness that to truly surrender involves a lot of letting go on all levels.

Let the wise guard their wandering thoughts
extremely subtle and difficult to perceive.
The thought that is well guarded
is the bearer of happiness.

The Buddha

NINETEEN
Letters from Students

Yoga and my cello playing

I feel that my cello playing has been enhanced and opened out by the cumulative, gradual influence of Yoga.

First, the ability to detach one's inner self and particularly one's breathing from the emotions and physical difficulties of playing mirrors the ability to breathe calmly whilst stretching one's limbs in Yoga.

Secondly, the balance and vitality of the spine growing naturally from sacrum to head, with relaxed and widening shoulder blades, is a vital component of cello playing and, I am sure, any physically challenging activity from tennis to Aikido, or dance to acrobatics.

David Waterman. (Cellist with the Endellion Quartet)

A letter from Scotland

Dearest Mina,

I wanted to tell you just how inspirational it has been for me to read your manuscript of 'The Distracted Centipede'. It has really helped me to push through my resistance to practising yoga on my own. Since reading it I have found myself leaping out of bed and getting down onto the floor to stretch and flex and re-attune with my body and, on a few rare occasions, my mind.

I realise that having been in the class with you as teacher is a big bonus. So many times, as my mind wanders off lord knows where, I hear your voice helping me to try and return to the breath.

Above all I feel that the book has put the ball firmly back in my own court. It is really helping me to begin to understand the difference between 'just doing yoga postures', or rediscovering my body and reuniting it with the other elements of myself.

For many years I haven't really lived in my body at all! Now I find that each day I discover yet another nook or cranny and try to just go with it...

My friend I just want to say a heart-felt thank you for putting down on paper what you do for us even more each Monday.

With love, Sally

When I do Yoga with Mina it's like she's clicked my 'refresh' button.

However tired, or achy, or emotionally down I am, I always come away calm and centred with Mina's words echoing in my ears; *'to continue that feeling in my everyday living'*. Concentrating on breathing and postures with Mina gently leading us is part of a miraculous renewal of the body and spirit. I can just let myself be and become detached from all my external worries, but at the same time be in charge of who I am. Also I feel more supple all the time and conscious of the limitless possibilities of exploring what my body can do, how it can extend and relax and even be turned on its head!

Yoga is fun and spiritual and endlessly revitalising. I gain energy from the rest of the group and always look forward to my 'fix' of Mina's Yoga.

Genista

Yoga and the art of cycling!

A couple of weeks ago, Fred and I went cycling. This was the first time for me in about five years. Fred goes much more regularly. After about ten minutes he said that he didn't like cycling with me because I went too fast. This was never the case in the past and I realise that it's because of the breathing exercises I'm learning with you in Yoga. Now I get out of breath much less than I ever have before.

Vanessa

' I've found my feet!'

After this morning's yoga session on 'standing with 100% enthusiasm in the feet', and for the first time in my life, I found my feet; there they were, right on the ground! Then I realised that when I was a tiny child and my mother was ill and couldn't sleep, I was warned, in no uncertain terms, to 'stop making a noise like a herd of elephants, and to *walk softly.*'

All my life I've been walking softly. Instead of letting the good earth carry my weight, I pulled myself up by my bootstraps from the scruff of my neck and, with my shoulders up to my ears, held my breath, tensing just about every other muscle and sinew in my body. And still my mother remained an insomniac!

The freedom I am now experiencing is a miracle.

Less awkward – more graceful

by poet, singer and, musician Christopher Twigg.

I noticed when I performed with my group, Chicken of the Woods, at the 12 Bar Club, that I felt more relaxed on stage, more present in my body. Time didn't seem to rush by so fast. I could play more accurately and listen better to what the others were doing, John on the double bass and Chris on the mandolin.

I felt under less pressure in awkward moments, like when I had to change the harmonica for a song in a different key or move the *capo* up and down. I felt more present to the audience and less fearful, more in touch with a sense of 'I am who I am and that is OK' and the best I can do. I had more control of the singing, a deeper sense of listening and hearing and the way I carried myself. The dignity of the great blues Masters like Muddy Waters, which has to do with authentic presence came to mind.

I find that Yoga gives me more trust in my body's memory so there is less need to keep looking to see what my hands are doing, which makes communication with the audience more intimate.

You asked me to say something about the 'negative' state I get into. What happens is that I lose interest and what was a feeling of delight in my body's balance becomes a thing of the past. The pleasure of feeling how my weight is going down my legs becomes so removed it just doesn't occur to me to feel.

I become preoccupied with ways to escape: alcohol, sex, dope, fantasies of travel. I wake with a hangover. I can still write stream of consciousness in that state of mind but Yoga seems unpleasant, it feels like I'm tuning in to my own alienation and discomfort.

Of course, when I make even a slight effort towards practising, maybe just lying on the carpet and feeling the contact and the texture of the rug, there is often a change towards feeling better again. To me it is the difference between 'being at home' or 'not at home with myself' or 'not at home'. It amazes me how quickly I forget the simplicity of the practice (breathing meditation for example) and get caught up in thrashing around with painful desires and bitter resentments to give up and, above all, to be unconscious.

Yoga brings me back to consciousness, to activity, to *INCORPORATION* – being in my body. Lines of F.G. Lorca from 'Poet in New York' come to mind where he says,

*'Despierta. Calla. Escucha. Incorporate un poco…
No solloces en sueños, amigo.'*

*'Wake up. Be silent. Listen. Come into your body a bit.
Don't sob in dreams, my friend.'*

So I become more embodied, more relaxed, more spacious, under less pressure, time seems to go more slowly. There is more enjoyment, feet on the ground, presence …less awkward, more graceful.

Yom Kippur – The Day of Atonement

'In years past I've found it too difficult to stay on my feet through the special standing prayers we recite on Yom Kippur, which can last up to two hours. I would always have to keep sitting down from time to time, to ease the pressure on my lower back.

Not so this year! I felt comfortable standing throughout. I was really pleased with myself and although it was out of keeping with Yom Kippur, I must confess, I felt rather smug. For I realised, having glanced around, that this achievement wasn't being matched by most of my fellow congregants, including the men. It made me appreciate the benefits and beauty of Yoga.

In my sixth decade I'd actually started learning to stand. It felt like a giant step forward.'

K.

'Paying more attention to the present'

I was introduced to Mina by my doctor after being diagnosed with arthritis in all my joints. After eight years it is not only that my pain is gone, my posture is better, I feel have been introduced to a new way of life altogether. Less thinking and being in my head, more paying attention to the present and living.

Bahar Fussell

Avoiding knee replacement surgery by getting to know my knees

Ten years ago I could hardly walk. My GP told me that there was nothing that could be done; once the knees go, that's it! She advised painkillers and the possibility of knee replacements when walking became impossible.

Lucky for me a couple of years after this doom-ridden prognosis I met Mina who told me she thought Yoga could help.

In fact it wasn't only painful knees I suffered from. For years I'd had crippling back trouble as well. Cranial osteopathy worked wonders but at least once a year I'd manage to 'put my back out' and need another series of treatments.

That's ten years ago. Today I have no pain in my knees, and occasional back pain responds almost miraculously to certain Yoga postures.

But it's not only Yoga postures that made the difference. Mina taught me that chronic physical pain is also a sign of deeply rooted childhood problems too painful to face up to, which recede into the subconscious and hide in strategic parts of our body.

Having been in psychotherapy for 15 years, despairing of ever being able to let go of certain experiences and also quite proud of the fact that 'I'd never really inhabited my body', I began to focus on these painful areas using Mina's imagery. The profound truth is that by working on releasing the tightly strung muscles I was also able to become aware of those early memories and in turn, release and let them go.

I believe that Mina's Yoga, is enabling me to incarnate properly at the age of 66! I also believe that perhaps by the time I'm 80 I'll be able to do a backbend! If more people lay down on the floor, taking the weight off their knees and hips each day, how much easier life would be for the overworked National Health Service!

TWENTY

Gratitude to teachers past and present

Namaste

What are we doing when we press our palms together and bow to each other in the Indian tradition?

> *I honour the place in you where the entire universe resides,*
> *I honour the place in you that is of love, of truth, of light, of peace.*
> *When you are in that place in you*
> *And I am in that place in me,*
> *We are truly present to each other.*

I would like to acknowledge the loving guidance of all my teachers in this difficult, ongoing process of awakening to authentic being.

Gratitude is a feeling that arises out of the depths of one's being. When it happens a glimpse of light appears, and we feel connected to all of life and feel part of it instead of isolated in our ego shell, made up of all our familiar likes and dislikes, fears, worries and preoccupations.

It is not necessary to belong to a religious sect, or to follow a guru to be devoted to God. The deepest devotion is to remember respect for life in all its forms and to feel love in our hearts.

I discovered that my pain and suffering come from not being able to slow down enough to experience this respect and thankfulness.

The more I practise the more I realise how much fortitude is required to stay on this inner path towards liberation. Respect and gratitude awaken towards those people, past and present, who have been inspiring examples guiding me to recognise the different stages and not become discouraged by difficulties and obstacles on the way.

The fact that they *all* said that it is difficult is somehow encouraging, as is the fact that they all said *'don't look to me, look within'*. Most of all it is being present and mindful of what is happening in our inner and outer world that is the true teacher and healer.

TWENTY ONE

Take it with two pinches of salt

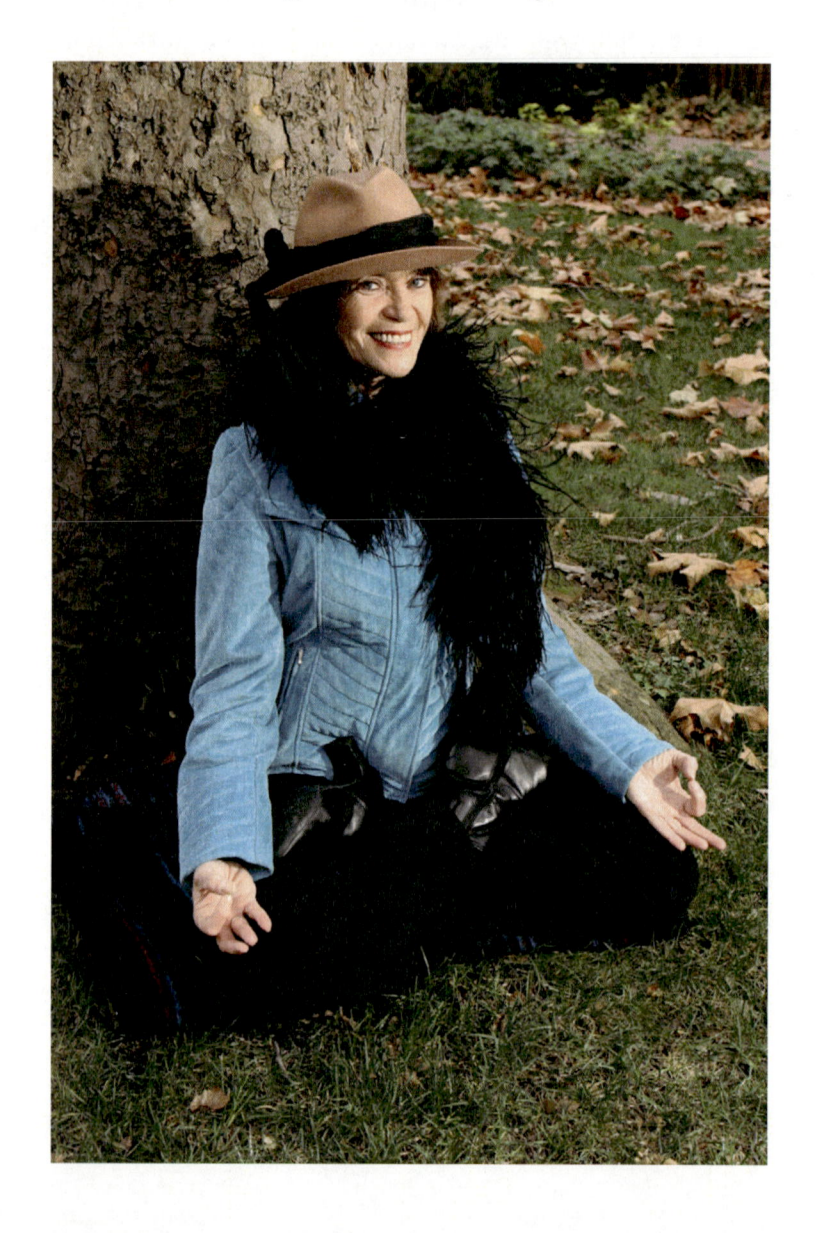

We need to question all 'authority' and all traditions and not just follow them blindly. 'Respectful irreverence' is what I mean by 'take it with two pinches of salt' With all due respect to teachers and teachings ...wake up, feel and think for yourself.

Listen to the silence in your heart
Find love within yourself
Make your body supple and co-ordinated
Keep your heart open.

'There are no good times around the corner.
There is only eternal now.
Only suckers put hope in the future.'
Alan Watts

There is life and light and joy and freshness yet.
May everyone enjoy good health and happiness.

Mina Semyon
London, 2004

About the Author

Mina Semyon was born in 1938 in the Soviet Union. She has been teaching Yoga for over 30 years. She was a student and friend of R.D.Laing, psychiatrist, poet, musician and spiritual teacher who initiated her on the path of awareness through the practice of Yoga and mindfulness. This, combined with an insistence of finding her authentic voice through the study of singing and sound with AntheaParashchak, has led to her unique way of teaching. In the process of transcending her harsh Russian childhood, what has evolved is a way of practising and teaching which incorporates our whole being - emotional, mental, physical and spiritual, in daily life and relationships. Her aim is to liberate the mind and body of everything that obscures the spirit of joy, love, compassion, spontaneity and playfulness. Mina appeared in the BBC television series and the book 'Every Body Knows' and the Yoga book 'Body Life' written by her ex-husband Arthur Balaskas. She is currently working on her life story 'You Don't Have to Die of Disappointment'.

Suggestions for further reading

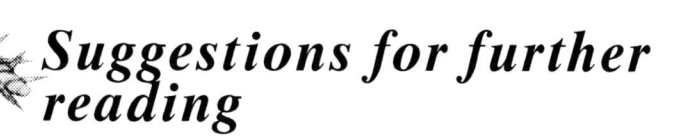

Thomas Moore
Care of the Soul: How to add depth and meaning to your every day life.
Judy Piatkus (Publishers) Ltd

Stephen Batchelor
Buddhism Without Belief: A Contemporary Guide to Awakening
London, Bloomsbury

Karfried Graf Von Durkheim
Hara: The vital Centre of Man
George Allen and Unwin

Lao Tsu
Tao Teh Ching
Translated by Gia-Fu Feng and Jane English
Wildwood House

The Essential Rumi
Translations by Coleman Barks with John Moyne
Castle Books

Gary Zukav
The Seat of the Soul
Simon & Schuster

The Essential Chogyam Trungpa
Shambhala

Bhagwan Shree Patanjali
Aphorisms of Yoga
Translated by Shree Purohit Swami with an introduction by
W.B. Yeats

The Bhagavad Gita
Penguin classics
Published by Penguin books
first published 1962

Pema Chodron
When things fall apart: heart advice for difficult times.
The places that scare you: A guide to fearlessness in difficult times.
Shambala Classics

Resources

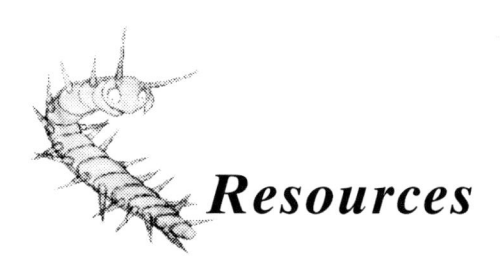

Mina Semyon

Self-Healing with Yoga and Mindfulness:
Workshops • Individual Sessions •
Regular Classes • Holidays

minasemyon@onetel.com
Phone: (0044) 020 7586 6593
FAX: (0044) 020 7328 2512

International R D Laing Institute
http://laingsociety.org/colloquia/inperson/minasemyon.htm

Dr Leon Redler, MD

Psychotherapist
0207 916 5191
leonredler@blueyonder.co.uk
Mediator
The Mediation Partnership
0207 916 7917
www.themediationpartnership.com
info@themediationpartnership.com
Author of diverse publications including
Just Listening: Ethics and Therapy (Xlibris, 2001) with Dr. Steven Gans
(with whom Dr Redler is involved in developing 'Just Listening' as an ethical-deconstructive therapy practice and teaching).
www.justlistening.com

Kira Balaskas

Thai Yoga Massage: How to use traditional Thai massage, yoga, and breathwork for healing and spiritual harmony.
Published by Thorsons 2002
website: www.thaiyogamassage.co.uk
email: info@thaiyogamassage.co.uk

Active Birth Centre

25 Bickerton Road
London N19 5JT
Tel: 020 7281 6760 - Fax: 020 7485 3503
www.activebirthcentre.com
jb@activebirthcentre.com

tel: 0207 2816760
fax: 0207 2638098
email: info@activebirthcentre.com
www.activebirthcentre.com

Books by Janet Balaskas

Preparing for Birth with Yoga: Thorsons.
New Active Birth: Thorsons.
Both available from www.activebirthcentre.com

ISBN 1-41202926-0